T0383347

Value-Based Care

Editor

LEE A. FLEISHER

ANESTHESIOLOGY CLINICS

www.anesthesiology.theclinics.com

Consulting Editor
LEE A. FLEISHER

December 2015 • Volume 33 • Number 4

ELSEVIER

1600 John F. Kennedy Boulevard • Suite 1800 • Philadelphia, Pennsylvania, 19103-2899

http://www.theclinics.com

ANESTHESIOLOGY CLINICS Volume 33, Number 4
December 2015 ISSN 1932-2275, ISBN-13: 978-0-323-40236-1

Editor: Patrick Manley
Developmental Editor: Kristen Helm

Anesthesiology Clinics (ISSN 1932-2275) is published quarterly by Elsevier Inc., 360 Park Avenue South, New York, NY 10010-1710. Months of issue are March, June, September, and December. Periodicals postage paid at New York, NY and at additional mailing offices. Subscription prices are $160.00 per year (US student/resident), $330.00 per year (US individuals), $400.00 per year (Canadian individuals), $533.00 per year (US institutions), $674.00 per year (Canadian institutions), $225.00 per year (Canadian and foreign student/resident), $455.00 per year (foreign individuals), and $674.00 per year (foreign institutions). To receive student and resident rate, orders must be accompanied by name of affiliated institution, date of term, and the *signature* of program/residency coordinator on institutions letterhead. Orders will be billed at individual rate until proof of status is received. Foreign air speed delivery is included in all *Clinics'* subscription prices. All prices are subject to change without notice. POSTMASTER: Send address changes to *Anesthesiology Clinics,* Elsevier Health Sciences Division, Subscription Customer Service, 3251 Riverport Lane, Maryland Heights, MO 63043. Customer Service (orders, claims, online, change of address): Elsevier Health Sciences Division, Subscription Customer Service, 3251 Riverport Lane, Maryland Heights, MO 63043. **Tel:1-800-654-2452 (U.S. and Canada); 314-447-8871 (outside U.S. and Canada). Fax: 314-447-8029. E-mail: journalscustomerservice-usa@elsevier. com (for print support); journalsonlinesupport-usa@elsevier.com (for online support).**

Reprints. For copies of 100 or more of articles in this publication, please contact the Commercial Reprints Department, Elsevier Inc., 360 Park Avenue South, New York, NY 10010-1710. Tel.: 212-633-3874; Fax: 212-633-3820; E-mail: reprints@elsevier.com.

Anesthesiology Clinics, is also published in Spanish by McGraw-Hill Inter-americana Editores S. A., P.O. Box 5-237, 06500 Mexico D. F., Mexico.

Anesthesiology Clinics, is covered in *MEDLINE/PubMed (Index Medicus), Current Contents/Clinical Medicine, Excerpta Medica, ISI/BIOMED,* and *Chemical Abstracts.*

Contributors

EDITOR

LEE A. FLEISHER, MD, FACC, FAHA
Robert D. Dripps Professor and Chair of Anesthesiology and Critical Care, Professor of Medicine, Perelman School of Medicine at the University of Pennsylvania, Philadelphia, Pennsylvania

AUTHORS

MICHAEL A. ASHBURN, MD, MPH
Professor, Department of Anesthesiology and Critical Care, University of Pennsylvania, Philadelphia, Pennsylvania

JOSHUA H. ATKINS, MD, PhD
Assistant Professor of Anesthesiology and Critical Care and Otorhinolaryngology Head and Neck Surgery, Department of Anesthesiology and Critical Care, Perelman School of Medicine of the University of Pennsylvania, Philadelphia, Pennsylvania

ARVIND CHANDRAKANTAN, MD, MBA, FAAP
Assistant Professor, Department of Anesthesiology, Stony Brook Medicine, Stony Brook, New York

BEVERLY CHANG, MD
Clinical Fellow, Department of Anesthesiology, Perioperative and Pain Medicine, Stanford University School of Medicine, Stanford, California

KATHERINE H. DOBIE, MD
Chief, Division of Ambulatory Anesthesiology; Assistant Professor of Anesthesiology, Department of Anesthesiology, Vanderbilt University School of Medicine, Nashville, Tennessee

PETER F. DUNN, MD
Executive Medical Director, Perioperative Services, Massachusetts General Hospital, Boston, Massachusetts

SUSAN L. FAGGIANI, RN, BA, CPHQ
Department of Anesthesiology, Weill Cornell Medical College, New York, New York

PETER M. FLEISCHUT, MD
Associate Professor, Department of Anesthesiology, Weill Cornell Medical College; Associate Chief Innovation Officer, NewYork-Presbyterian Hospital, New York, New York

LEE A. FLEISHER, MD, FACC, FAHA
Robert D. Dripps Professor and Chair of Anesthesiology and Critical Care, Professor of Medicine, Perelman School of Medicine at the University of Pennsylvania, Philadelphia, Pennsylvania

CAROLINE D. FOSNOT, DO, MS
Assistant Professor of Clinical Anesthesiology, Department of Anesthesiology and Critical Care, Hospital of University Pennsylvania, Perelman School of Medicine at the University of Pennsylvania, Philadelphia, Pennsylvania

TONG JOO GAN, MD, MHS, FRCA
Professor and Chairman, Department of Anesthesiology, Stony Brook University School of Medicine, Stony Brook, New York

GREGORY P. GIAMBRONE, MS
Staff Associate, Department of Anesthesiology, Weill Cornell Medical College, New York, New York

MICHAEL P.W. GROCOTT, BSc, MBBS, MD, FRCA, FRCP, FFICM
Professor, Integrative Physiology and Critical Illness Group, Clinical and Experimental Sciences, Faculty of Medicine, University Hospital Southampton NHS Foundation Trust, NIHR Respiratory Biomedical Research Centre, University of Southampton, Southampton, Hampshire; NIAA Health Services Research Centre, Royal College of Anaesthetists; UCLH Surgical Outcomes Research Centre, UCL Centre for Anaesthesia, London, United Kingdom

JAMES R. HEBL, MD
Professor, Department of Anesthesiology, Mayo Clinic, Rochester, Minnesota

JOSEPH A. HYDER, MD, PhD
Assistant Professor, Division of Critical Care Medicine, Department of Anesthesiology, Kern Center for the Science of Health Care Delivery, Mayo Clinic, Rochester, Minnesota

KEITH A. JONES, MD
Department of Anesthesiology and Perioperative Medicine, Alfred Habeeb Professor and Chair, University of Alabama at Birmingham, Birmingham, Alabama

JOHN KEOGH, MD
Associate Professor, Department of Anesthesiology and Critical Care; Director of Perelman Center for Advanced Medicine, Perelman School of Medicine at the University of Pennsylvania, Philadelphia, Pennsylvania

JEFFREY R. KIRSCH, MD
Professor and Chair, Associate Dean for Clinical and Veterans Affairs, Department of Anesthesiology and Perioperative Medicine, Oregon Health and Science University, Portland, Oregon

WILTON C. LEVINE, MD
Associate Medical Director, Perioperative Services, Massachusetts General Hospital, Boston, Massachusetts

JAVIER LORENZO, MD
Clinical Instructor, Department of Anesthesiology, Perioperative and Pain Medicine, Stanford University School of Medicine, Stanford, California

ALEX MACARIO, MD, MBA
Vice-Chair for Education, Program Director, Anesthesia Residency; Professor, Departments of Anesthesiology, Perioperative and Pain Medicine and Health Research and Policy, Stanford University School of Medicine, Stanford, California

MICHAEL G. MYTHEN, MBBS, MD, FRCA, FFICM, FFAI(Hon)
Professor, NIAA Health Services Research Centre, Royal College of Anaesthetists; UCLH Surgical Outcomes Research Centre, UCL Centre for Anaesthesia; UCLH/UCL NIHR Biomedical Research Centre, London, United Kingdom

PETER PRYZBYLKOWSKI, MD
Assistant Professor, Department of Anesthesiology and Critical Care, University of Pennsylvania, Philadelphia, Pennsylvania

STEPHEN T. ROBINSON, MD
Clinical Professor and Vice Chair for Clinical Anesthesia, Department of Anesthesiology and Perioperative Medicine, Oregon Health and Science University, Portland, Oregon

WARREN S. SANDBERG, MD, PhD
Chair, Department of Anesthesiology, Professor of Anesthesiology, Surgery and Biomedical Informatics, Vanderbilt University School of Medicine, Nashville, Tennessee

TIFFANY TEDORE, MD
Associate Professor; Co-Director of Regional Anesthesiology and Acute Pain Medicine, Department of Anesthesiology, Weill Cornell Medical College, New York, New York

VIKRAM TIWARI, MBA, PhD
Director of Perioperative Analytics, Department of Anesthesiology, Vanderbilt University Hospital; Assistant Professor of Anesthesiology, Vanderbilt University School of Medicine, Nashville, Tennessee

THOMAS R. VETTER, MD, MPH
Department of Anesthesiology and Perioperative Medicine, Maurice S. Albin Professor and Vice Chair, University of Alabama at Birmingham, Birmingham, Alabama

RONIEL WEINBERG, MD
Assistant Professor; Co-Director of Regional Anesthesiology and Acute Pain Medicine, Department of Anesthesiology, Weill Cornell Medical College, New York, New York

LISA WITKIN, MD
Assistant Professor, Department of Anesthesiology, Weill Cornell Medical College, New York, New York

Contents

> Perioperative medicine describes the practice of patient centered, multi-disciplinary, and integrated medical care of patients from the moment of contemplation of surgery until full recovery. The value proposition for perioperative medicine rests on defining benefits that outweigh the costs of change. This article discusses the concept of value in the context of healthcare and highlights a number of reasons for relative market failure. Five key opportunities for adding value in the perioperative journey are suggested: collaborative decision-making, lifestyle modification before surgery, standardization of in-hospital perioperative care, achieving full recovery after surgery, and the use of data for quality improvement.

> An enhanced recovery after surgery strategy will be increasingly adopted in the era of value-based care. The various elements in each enhanced recovery after surgery protocol are likely to add value to the overall patient surgical journey. Although the evidence varies considerably based on type of surgery and patient group, the team-based approach of care should be universally applied to patient care. This article provides an overview of up-to-date techniques and methodology for enhanced recovery, including an overview of value-based care, delivery, and the evidence base supporting enhanced recovery after surgery.

> Health care costs continue to increase, and the approach of countries and insurers is to focus on the value of the care delivered. Value is a function of quality in relation to costs. The perspective of the individual measuring value is important. Calculation of costs may include return to work if the employer's perspective is taken. The patients' perspectives include out-of-pocket expenses and work lost for both patients and potentially caregivers. The authors provide one example in the area of sleep apnea in which the anesthesiologist can provide value uniquely by being part of the team making the diagnosis.

Consolidation in anesthesiology practice and the rest of health care creates pressure to improve the product offered by anesthesia professionals. Anesthesia professionals must offer more than a reliable stream of anesthetized, operated, and recovered patients to remain competitive. By pooling resources and application of leadership effort, large departments and group practices can conduct individual-level value assessments of clinicians. Individual clinicians can be incentivized to improve their personal value proposition. By creating an interlocking program of ongoing assessment, career development coaching and opportunities, as well as compensation, departments and group practices can return value to individual clinicians by curating and accelerating their career and capability development.

Anesthesiologists are obligated to demonstrate the value of the care they provide. The Centers for Medicare and Medicaid Services has multiple performance-based payment programs to drive high-value care and motivate integrated care for surgical patients and hospitalized patients. These programs rely on diverse arrays of performance measures and complex reporting rules. Among all specialties, anesthesiology has tremendous potential to effect wide-ranging change on diverse measures. Performance measures deserve scrutiny by anesthesiologists as tools to improve care, the means by which payment is determined, and as a means to demonstrate the value of care to surgeons, hospitals, and patients.

This article reviews the management of an operating room (OR) schedule and use of the schedule to add value to an organization. We review the methodology of an OR block schedule, daily OR schedule management, and post anesthesia care unit patient flow. We discuss the importance of a well-managed OR schedule to ensure smooth patient care, not only in the OR, but throughout the entire hospital.

Lean strategies can be readily applied to health care in general and operating rooms specifically. The emphasis is on the patient as the customer, respect and engagement of all providers, and leadership from management. The strategy of lean is to use continuous improvement to eliminate waste from the care process, leaving only value-added activities. This iterative process progressively adds the steps of identifying the 7 common forms of waste (transportation, inventory, motion, waiting, overproduction, overprocessing, and defects), 5S (sort, simplify, sweep, standardize, sustain), visual controls, just-in-time processing, level-loaded work, and built-in quality to achieve the highest quality of patient care.

Ambulatory anesthesia's popularity continues to increase and techniques continue to adapt to the needs of patients. Alterations in existing medications are promising. Postoperative nausea and vomiting, pain, obstructive sleep apnea, and chronic comorbidities are concerns in ambulatory settings. Regional anesthesia has multiple advantages over general anesthesia. The implementation of the Affordable Health Care Act specifically affects ambulatory settings as the demand and need for patients to undergo screening procedures with anesthesia. The question remains what the best strategy is to meet the needs of our future patients while preserving economic feasibility within an already strained health care system.

Effective and efficient acute pain management strategies have the potential to improve medical outcomes, enhance patient satisfaction, and reduce costs. Pain management records are having an increasing influence on patient choice of health care providers and will affect future financial reimbursement. Dedicated acute pain and regional anesthesia services are invaluable in improving acute pain management. In addition, nonpharmacologic and alternative therapies, as well as information technology, should be viewed as complimentary to traditional pharmacologic treatments commonly used in the management of acute pain. The use of innovative technologies to improve acute pain management may be worthwhile for health care institutions.

As health care costs threaten the economic stability of American society, increasing pressures to focus on value-based health care have led to the development of protocols for fast-track cardiac surgery and for delirium management. Critical care services can be led by anesthesiologists with the goal of improving ICU outcomes and at the same time decreasing the rising cost of ICU medicine.

Healthcare delivery and payment systems in the United States must continue to be reformed to address currently untenably increasing healthcare expenditures, while increasing the quality of care. The Perioperative Surgical Home is a highly patient-centered approach to care, focusing on the standardization, coordination, transitions, and value of care throughout the perioperative continuum, including after hospital discharge. To increase the value of surgical care, any Perioperative Surgical Home model must translate, implement, and sustain improvements in quality, safety, and satisfaction, plus cost reduction strategies, throughout the perioperative continuum. Healthcare informatics, analytics, decision support, and practice change are central to this effort.

Chronic pain affects an estimated 100 million people a year in the United States and costs society anywhere from $560 to $635 billion annually. The patient-centered medical home and the patient-centered medical home-neighbor models of care have been advocated to improve patient outcomes. These models of care advocate improved coordination of care within the primary care and specialty care setting. The authors present the patient-centered medical home model of care and suggest how this model of care might be used to improve patient outcomes for patients with chronic pain.

ANESTHESIOLOGY CLINICS

THE CLINICS ARE AVAILABLE ONLINE!
Access your subscription at:
www.theclinics.com

Erratum

In the March 2015 issue of *Anesthesiology Clinics* (Volume 33, Issue 1), in the article "Pathophysiology of Major Surgery and the Role of Enhanced Recovery Pathways and the Anesthesiologist to Improve Outcomes" by Michael J. Scott and Timothy E. Miller, the source of Figure 1 was excluded from the figure legend. Figure 1 originally appeared in *Critical Care Clinics* (Volume 26, Issue 3) in the article "Enhanced Recovery After Surgery: The Future of Improving Surgical Care" by Krishna K. Varadhan, Dileep N. Lobo, and Olle Ljungqvist.

http://dx.doi.org/10.1016/j.anclin.2015.10.001
1932-2275/15/$ – see front matter
anesthesiology.theclinics.com

Preface

Value—The Current Cure for Health Care's Ailments?

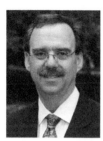

Lee A. Fleisher, MD, FACC, FAHA
Editor

Over the past several years, there has been a concerted effort to focus on value in health care as a means of driving improvement. Value is defined as the quality of care or outcome divided by the cost of delivering that care. Michael Porter of the Harvard Business School has tried to focus attention on this concept as a means of aligning the different stakeholders in achieving the triple aim of better care, lower costs, and better health of the population.[1,2] Anesthesiology has come to this party later than some other specialties but has recently focused on the drive to demonstrate value to our patients, the players, and society in general. Projects such as the Perioperative Surgical Home are among the group of activities centered around the value proposition. Pain management and critical care have also been areas in which anesthesiologists have focused their attention. Thomas Lee, of Press-Ganey and Partners Healthcare, and I have recently written a perspective on how anesthesiologists can impact the value proposition in health care.[3] In trying to create an issue of *Anesthesiology Clinics* devoted to value, I have attempted to look at both the United States and England for leaders who have focused attention on different areas within our traditional and nontraditional purview to provide insights into how best to demonstrate those areas in which we can impact outcomes and costs. I hope this issue will provide a roadmap to help us achieve the goal of the triple aim.

Lee A. Fleisher, MD, FACC, FAHA
Perelman School of Medicine
University of Pennsylvania
Philadelphia, PA 19104, USA

E-mail address:
Lee.fleisher@uphs.upenn.edu

Anesthesiology Clin 33 (2015) xv–xvi
http://dx.doi.org/10.1016/j.anclin.2015.08.001
1932-2275/15/$ – see front matter © 2015 Published by Elsevier Inc.
anesthesiology.theclinics.com

REFERENCES

1. Porter ME. A strategy for health care reform—toward a value-based system. New Engl J Med 2009;361(2):109–12.
2. Porter ME. What is value in health care? New Engl J Med 2010;363(26):2477–81.
3. Fleisher LA, Lee TH. Anesthesiology and anesthesiologists in the era of value-driven health care. Healthc (Amst) 2015;3(2):63–6.

Perioperative Medicine: The Value Proposition for Anesthesia?
A UK Perspective on Delivering Value from Anesthesiology

Michael P.W. Grocott, BSc, MBBS, MD, FRCA, FRCP, FFICM[a,b,c,]*,
Michael G. Mythen, MBBS, MD, FRCA, FFICM[b,c,d]

KEYWORDS

- Perioperative medicine • Perioperative physician • Anesthesiology • Anesthesia
- Value • Value proposition • Health economics • Cost-effectiveness

KEY POINTS

- Perioperative medicine is a patient-focused, multidisciplinary, and integrated approach to delivering the best possible health care throughout the perioperative journey from the moment of contemplation of surgery until full recovery.
- Perioperative medicine offers a physician-led vision of perioperative care in the twenty-first century and beyond. It extends the roles of the anesthetist beyond the operating room/theater into the wider hospital and community role and defines care delivery around the patient (as partner or consumer) rather than the care providers.
- Value considerations in health care in general, and perioperative medicine in particular, are complicated by the difficulty of attaching a monetary value to health outcomes, such as survival or freedom from disability.

Continued

[a] Integrative Physiology and Critical Illness Group, Clinical and Experimental Sciences, Faculty of Medicine, University of Southampton / Anaesthesia and Critical Care Research Unit, University Hospital Southampton NHS Foundation Trust / Southampton NIHR Respiratory Biomedical Research Centre, University of Southampton, Room CE.93, Mailpoint 24, Tremona Road, Southampton, Hampshire SO16 6YD, UK; [b] NIAA Health Services Research Centre, Royal College of Anaesthetists, Red Lion Square, London, WC1R 4SG, UK; [c] UCLH Surgical Outcomes Research Centre / UCLH/UCL NIHR Biomedical Research Centre, London, University College London Hospitals NHS Foundation Trust, 149 Tottenham Court Road, London, W1T 7DN, UK; [d] Centre for Anaesthesia, UCL, Gower Street, London, WC1E 6BT, UK
* Corresponding author. Integrative Physiology and Critical Illness Group, Clinical and Experimental Sciences, Faculty of Medicine, University of Southampton / Anaesthesia and Critical Care Research Unit, University Hospital Southampton NHS Foundation Trust / Southampton NIHR Respiratory Biomedical Research Centre, University of Southampton, Room CE.93, Mailpoint 24, Tremona Road, Southampton, Hampshire SO16 6YD, UK.
E-mail address: mike.grocott@soton.ac.uk

Anesthesiology Clin 33 (2015) 617–628
http://dx.doi.org/10.1016/j.anclin.2015.07.003
1932-2275/15/$ – see front matter © 2015 Elsevier Inc. All rights reserved.
anesthesiology.theclinics.com

Continued

- The value proposition for perioperative medicine is based on the efficient reapplication of current resources, rather than through major new investment. All the elements of perioperative medicine have been implemented somewhere, but few if any centers have successfully implemented the complete package of perioperative care.
- The successful implementation of the Enhanced Recovery Partnership Programme in England suggests that such projects can be implemented at minimal cost with increased productivity and quality through the application of leadership and quality improvement techniques.

INTRODUCTION

Perioperative medicine describes the practice of patient-centered, multidisciplinary, and integrated medical care of patients from the moment of contemplation of surgery until full recovery.[1,2] The Royal College of Anaesthetists has expressed a commitment to "developing a collaborative programme for the delivery of perioperative care across the UK" and to leading the development of UK perioperative medicine.[3] The Perioperative Surgical Home is a similar initiative led by the American Society of Anesthesiologists in the United States and embraces a parallel vision of physician-led seamless patient-centered care through the surgical pathway from shared decision making to full recovery.[4]

Economics and health care make uncomfortable bedfellows in 2015. In the aftermath of the global financial crisis, cost containment is a dominant theme in an economic environment in which health care demand continues to increase and government budgets are tight. Surgical interventions are costly, particularly in the developed world where a substantial proportion of the health care infrastructure and labor force is focused on delivering elective surgery as safely as possible, often within large well-equipped hospitals. Furthermore, it is likely that the volume (and therefore aggregate cost) of surgery, both at a national and global level, will increase with time because of several interacting factors predominantly related to demographic change.

Health economics is commonly recognized as a special case within general economics because of a variety of factors that result in relative market failure.[5] One important factor in this regard is uncertainty about whether a monetary value can be attached to health-related benefits, such as longer life or being free of disability. As a consequence, many considerations of value in relation to health care are presented in relative terms, rather than using absolute monetary units. It is in this context that the general value proposition for perioperative medicine must be justified.

This article outlines some key elements of the health care economic landscape including consideration of the reasons for relative market failure. It then explores some concepts of value in health care, describes the scope of perioperative medicine, and explores the assertion that perioperative medicine offers a value proposition to health care systems, purchasers, policy makers, patients, and the public, with specific reference to the UK health care environment.

HEALTH CARE DELIVERY IS RESOURCE CONSTRAINED

Definitions of the dismal science have evolved since Adam Smith[6] described economics as "an inquiry into the nature and causes of the wealth of nations" in 1776. A more useful formulation defines economics as "the science that studies human behavior as a relationship between ends and scarce means that have alternative uses."[7] In other words, economics is the study of choice when resources are constrained.

In practical terms, there are limits on the available resources in almost any human context. In health care, the combination of relentless growth in demand in an environment of constrained financial resources inevitably leads to increasingly difficult choices. During the 50 years from 1960 to 2010, overall spending on health care increased from 5.1% to 17.6% of gross domestic product (GDP) in the United States, from 5.4% to 11.4% in Canada, and from 3.9% to 9.6% in the United Kingdom.[8] Such levels of growth are not sustainable indefinitely. The future trajectory of health care spending is uncertain because of the profound tensions between essentially limitless demand (as we strive to extend the quality and quantity of life), a limited and uncertain overall government spending envelope, and competing calls on government and private spending.

The United States provides a particular example of progressive growth in health care expenditure (as a proportion of GDP) in what has been an uncontrolled market. US Congressional Budget Office extrapolation of historical data leads to the prediction that health care expenditure will reach 98.9% of US GDP in 2082 (based on the untenable assumption that current policies are maintained).[9] When assumptions reflecting limits to excess cost growth are incorporated, the predicted GDP proportion for health care still approaches 50% by 2082.[9] Such outcomes are unlikely to be palatable to the voting public, which leads to the conclusion that tough decisions about resource allocation and cost containments in health care are inevitable in the coming years and that critical analysis of the relative value of different health care approaches is important. It follows that the definition and demonstration of value are a core priority for all those with an interest in delivering the best health outcomes to patients, communities, and nations.

HEALTH CARE ECONOMICS AND MARKET FAILURE

Health economics is generally considered to be a special case within economics because a variety of factors contribute to relative market failure. These factors include the magnitude of government intervention, inevitable uncertainties, asymmetric information, high barriers to entry, externalities, and the involvement of third-party agents.[5] The following paragraph explains each of these factors in turn.

Although the level of government intervention varies between nations, the phenomenon of government involvement can be considered a universal factor within health care markets and inevitably leads to distortions in price-setting behavior. Profound uncertainties exist on both sides of the cost-benefit equation in the health care market. For example, uncertainty may exist in relation to the efficacy (benefit) of a particular treatment in a specific patient. More strikingly, uncertainties in quantifying benefits, in relation to the true value of human life and the relative values of different levels of quality of life are likely unresolvable.[10] Even in relation to their own life, such judgments differ between individuals and within individuals at different times and under different conditions during their life span.

The challenges of attributing a monetary equivalent to these fundamentally important personal benefits contribute to the difficulty in describing value in the context of health care. Asymmetric information is a consequence of the disparity in knowledge between physicians and patients. Although the involvement of well-informed patients with chronic conditions in their own care decisions is reducing this factor in some clinical areas, this phenomenon is uncommon in the perioperative setting. High barriers to entry exist because of the costs of credentialing at several stages in the development of independent medical practitioners (from medical school to postgraduate diplomas). Such barriers to entry can be seen as a means of ensuring quality within the medical work force or, alternatively, may be viewed as a factor leading to artificial elevation of provider (doctor) prices in the health care marketplace. An externality is a cost or benefit that affects a party that did not choose to incur that cost of benefit.[11] Examples of (negative) externalities in health care include antimicrobial resistance as a consequence of indiscriminate prescription of antibiotics or the effects of second-hand smoke on passive smokers. Taken together, all these factors militate against the function of an effective market and add complexity to the definition of value in the context of health care.

DEFINING VALUE IN HEALTH CARE

The notion of value relates to the relationship between cost and benefit in a transaction or financial decision. By definition, the customer defines value. Although price is defined by the monetary amount that customer and provider can agree on at the time of a transaction (ie, defined by both parties to the transaction), value is defined by the customers perception of benefit.

Definitions of value use various approaches to describing the relationship between costs and benefits for any particular purchasing decision and are commonly expressed in monetary units. Arguably the simplest way of expressing this relationship is the simple business formula[12]:

Value = Benefits − Cost

An alternative approach proposed for evaluation of health care decisions considers benefits as a proportion of cost[13]:

Value = Benefit/Cost

A fundamental limitation for such definitions of value in the health care setting is the difficulty in attaching a monetary equivalent to health care outcomes (see earlier discussion). Inability to quantify (in monetary terms) the benefit component of the cost-benefit relationship limits any assessment of absolute value. Consequently, relative approaches to value using non-monetary metrics may provide a useful if imperfect alternative.

Several more sophisticated approaches to considering the notion of a value proposition have been applied to the context of assessing value in health care, including cost-effectiveness analysis, cost-utility analysis, and incremental cost-effectiveness ratios (ICERs) (**Box 1**).[14] However, through describing the incremental cost associated with an individual unit of effect (health care benefit), ICERs come back to attributing a monetary equivalent to a health outcome. From a policy perspective, this has led to significant concerns that such approaches will inevitably lead to health rationing. Although some form of rationing (controlled allocation of scarce resource) is inevitable in a resource-constrained health care environment, the notion that this occurs is considered unacceptable by some policy makers. The 2010 Patient Protection and Affordable Care Act in the United States explicitly forbids the use of disability discounted life measures to make decisions about the relative value of different health care approaches.[15] Conversely, the National Institute for Health and Care Excellence in the United Kingdom explicitly uses ICERs in relation to threshold willingness to pay values.[16]

A simple conceptual approach commonly used in health care is the cost-effectiveness matrix (**Fig. 1**).[17] This approach facilitates identification of innovations at extremes of the value spectrum and suggests adoption (category 4, southeast quadrant) where effectiveness is improved and costs are reduced or rejection (category 1,

---

Box 1
Value metrics in relation to health care

Cost minimization analysis is a method of comparing different approaches that use comparisons of costs when benefits have been shown to be equivalent (eg, interventions have equivalent effectiveness).

Cost-benefit (benefit-cost) analysis is a method of comparing different approaches that present both costs and benefits as monetary values. Owing to the difficulty of attributing monetary value to health outcomes, this approach is usually considered to have substantial limitations in the context of health care value.

Cost-effectiveness analysis (CEA) is a method of comparing different approaches that use comparisons of relative costs and benefits.

Cost-utility analysis (CUA) is a special case of CEA whereby benefits are expressed in terms of number of years in full health or full health discounted by a factor (such as quality of life or disability).

Incremental cost-effectiveness ratio (ICER) is the difference in cost between 2 approaches, described in monetary units, divided by the difference in effect, described in terms of health outcomes:

$$ICER = (C_1-C_0)/(E_1-E_0)$$

The ICER is the incremental cost associated with an individual unit of effect.

Using ICER in cost-effectiveness analysis in health care results in the attribution of monetary cost to health outcomes. In the specific case in which ICER is used in CUA, the result is the attribution of a monetary cost to an adjusted survival outcome (eg, quality-adjusted life years).

Data from Jolicoeur LM, Jones-Grizzle AJ, Boyer JG. Guidelines for performing a pharmacoeconomic analysis. Am J Hosp Pharm 1992;49(7):1741–7.

---

northwest quadrant) when the reverse pattern occurs. However, in many cases, this approach does not resolve value uncertainty or provide a solution to questions of relative value for innovations that fall within the same category. Opportunities for adding value may arise from achieving the same level of effectiveness using less resource (south) or through achieving less effectiveness with a greater proportional reduction in cost (category 3, southwest), thereby freeing up resources for alternative uses.

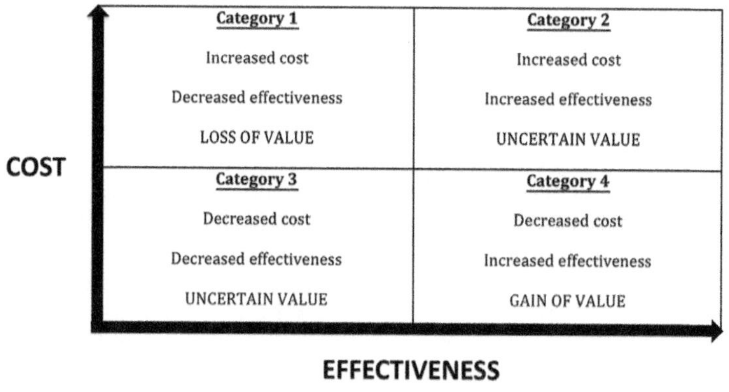

	Category 1	Category 2
	Increased cost	Increased cost
	Decreased effectiveness	Increased effectiveness
	LOSS OF VALUE	UNCERTAIN VALUE
COST	Category 3	Category 4
	Decreased cost	Decreased cost
	Decreased effectiveness	Increased effectiveness
	UNCERTAIN VALUE	GAIN OF VALUE

EFFECTIVENESS

Fig. 1. Simple matrix relating cost, effectiveness, and value.

WHY FOCUS ON VALUE?

Maximizing value equates to the achievement of the most possible benefit per unit cost,[13] that is, the efficient delivery of health care with respect to financial resources. Framed in these terms, the goal of maximizing value should be of the top priority to all stakeholders in the delivery and receipt of health care, given the context of an inevitably resource-limited environment. Maximizing value contributes to the sustainability of health care overall and therefore benefits individual patients and populations of patients (communities, nations) as well as providers and policy makers.

Given that value is defined by customer needs, rather than provider characteristics, it follows that value should be measured across a patient pathway, rather than in relation to a component of that pathway.[13] Focusing on inputs (costs) and outputs (benefits = patient outcomes) at a practitioner or departmental level obscures the true relationship from a customer (patient) perspective. For the same reasons, value should be estimated across the full cycle of care, rather than over shorter episodes during that cycle.[13] Maximizing value in the delivery of surgical services is therefore achieved by focusing on the whole patient journey: the pathway of delivered care and the ultimate outcomes of interest to the patient. The patient-centered, integrated, and multidisciplinary focus of perioperative medicine aligns perfectly with this approach.

Several results follow from an approach to health care focused on maximizing value through attention to cost and outcomes across the whole patient pathway.[13] First, accountability for value must be shared across professional and administrative boundaries, including between hospital and the community. Second, reimbursement must be aligned with value, either at an individual or institutional level, to avoid perverse incentives that drive behaviors toward nonproductive processes and practices that result in reduced efficiency and failure to maximize patient benefit. Third, cost reduction within a component of a pathway (eg, department) may be counterproductive unless viewed within the context of the delivery of benefit by the whole pathway. Fourth, the measurement reporting and comparison of outcomes to drive quality improvement is essential to improving value. Finally, the feedback loops that drive quality improvement have limited utility unless the end result is measured: process refinement is a means to an end, rather than an end in itself.

DEFINING PERIOPERATIVE MEDICINE

Perioperative medicine describes the practice of patient-centered, multidisciplinary, and integrated medical care of patients from the moment of contemplation of surgery until fill recovery.[1] The 2 key elements of this definition are the temporal scope and the patient-centered focus. The temporal span of perioperative medicine extends from the moment that surgery is first contemplated, when the benefits and risks of undergoing surgery can be evaluated and patients and clinicians can engage in a process of shared, or collaborative, decision making. The scope extends through to complete recovery or, in some cases, failure of recovery and death.

Patient centered is in many ways the opposite of doctor or clinician centered: care is defined by the patients' journey through the medical system, not by the practitioners and teams that interact with the patient during this journey or by the environment in which they work. Inevitably, such patient-centered care is multidisciplinary and integrated; the artificial barriers that separate primary and secondary care, or different professional groupings such as surgeons, anesthesiologists, or physiotherapists, become secondary to the delivery of care that delivers the best outcome for the patient.

WHAT CONSTITUTES PERIOPERATIVE MEDICINE

The constituent elements of perioperative medicine follow logically from the definitions offered in the previous section. Thus, before surgery, perioperative medicine encompasses preoperative risk evaluation, collaborative (shared) decision making about the primary surgical procedure and any adjunctive therapies,[1] optimization of all aspects of physiologic function before surgery through lifestyle modification (exercise/activity, weight loss, smoking and alcohol reduction),[18–20] and optimizing the management of long-term health problems (comorbidities) to minimize the risk of adverse outcome during or after surgery. In the intraoperative phase, it encompasses individualized goal-directed optimal intraoperative care across the full spectrum of perioperative interventions but critically care that is standardized and consistently delivered to the highest quality through process mapping and monitored delivery with inbuilt quality improvement mechanisms.

After surgery, the appropriate level of postoperative care both within hospital and after discharge should be targeted to the defined needs of individual patients based on the type of surgery and their personal resilience profile.[1] Finally, this care should be continued until full recovery and should encompass rehabilitation to best possible function as well as reevaluation and management of long-term conditions and appropriate management of any incidental health problems.[1] When full recovery is not achievable, the pathway should result in the best care possible for those left with disability or long-term conditions, including appropriate end-of-life care.

Finally, the entire perioperative journey may be one of few contacts that an individual patient has with health care professionals and therefore offers opportunities for perioperative physicians and other members of the perioperative care team to contribute to health improvement through general health messaging as well as primary, secondary, and tertiary preventative strategies, not limited to the condition under treatment from surgery.[1] The preoperative period offers a unique opportunity to invest in improving physiologic function in a short defined period, for example, through physical prehabilitation, in patients who are likely to be highly motivated in the face of an imminent personal threat.[18]

PERIOPERATIVE MEDICINE IN THE UNITED KINGDOM

The delivery of health care in general, and perioperative medicine in particular, in the United Kingdom provides an interesting example of the relationship between value and cost in health care. International comparisons suggest that largely unified health care systems (eg, United Kingdom) outperform countries without universal health insurance coverage (eg, United States) in terms of quality, access, efficiency, and equity.[21] The vast majority of health care within the United Kingdom is provided by the National Health Service (NHS) and paid for out of general taxation. The NHS was founded in 1948, based on 3 core principles: that it meet the needs of everyone, that it be free at the point of delivery, and that it be based on clinical need, not the ability to pay.[22] Thus, for the vast majority of health care delivered in the United Kingdom, there is a single payer and single provider and a shared belief in a set of core principles. Providers receive nationally determined bundled payments (with minor adjustments to reflect regional economies).

At a hospital (or hospital group) level, providers compete in a limited internal market with increasing potential over time for redistribution of work (ie, elective surgical cases) by commissioners of health care who are the agents of the payer (the Government dispersing taxpayer money). Commissioners demand value for money, and this is determined by a simple quality:cost equation, which has resulted in the pursuit of quality as the principle driver of providers. Volume is not necessarily good business and usually not in the patients' or societies' interests. Wrong surgery in the wrong patient is always a bad and expensive outcome from which no one gains. Providers who deliver high-quality outcomes, and thus value, in general have better balanced books and happier staff as a result of a job well done and a better working environment; this is a value not volume market. High complication rates and readmissions wreck budgets and reduce morale. An added advantage of the single-payer system is the consistency of expectations and rewards and reduction in friction costs (eg, the administration of complex multipayer systems). The Enhanced Recovery Partnership Programme was a national perioperative implementation project within the NHS (in England) that demonstrated the advantages of such a system (**Box 2**).[23,24]

Box 2
Case study: UK Enhanced Recovery Partnership Programme

Background

Enhanced recovery or fast-track surgery programs were well established in a small number of UK NHS hospitals by 2009. These hospitals had some of the best results in the system, with high levels of patient satisfaction, fewer complications, shorter lengths of hospital stay, and low readmission rates.

Short history

The UK Department of Health's Enhanced Recovery Partnership Programme ran from May 2009 to May 2012 with the aim of achieving the rapid spread and adoption of Enhanced Surgical Recovery in England. Major colorectal, orthopedic, gynecologic, and urologic surgeries were chosen for national implementation. The objective was to embed emergency room teams and principles throughout the system and deliver the same value offered by the best 10% of institutions at the outset (higher patient satisfaction at reduced cost).

Cost of program

Despite an increase in productivity (the number of elective cases performed per annum), net savings estimated to be in excess of $50 million per annum were reported by the end of year 2. Modest national investments were made in leadership teams, change management experts, meetings, and materials (implementation guides, Web sites, audit tools). This result was mirrored regionally and locally. Most programs reported in a year recovery of investment.

Benefits

Patients in the Enhanced Recovery Partnership Programme reported very high (>90%) levels of satisfaction, considerably higher than national benchmarks. National data for England (Hospital Episode Statistics) demonstrated increased productivity and reduced lengths of stay to target levels set at the median of the best 10% of institutions at the start. There was no increase in readmission rates. Net financial savings were mirrored by freeing up 170,000 bed days per annum.

A consensus statement signed by 17 of the UK's health care leaders in April 2012 (3 years after start), including the NHS Medical Director and presidents of the Royal Colleges of Anaesthetists, Physicians, and Surgeons, concludes: "We believe that enhanced recovery should now be considered as standard practice for most patients undergoing major surgery across a range of procedures and specialties."

Data from Mythen MG. Spread and adoption of enhanced recovery from elective surgery in the English National Health Service. Can J Anaesth 2015;62(2):105–9; and Simpson JC, Moonesinghe SR, Grocott MP, et al; National Enhanced Recovery Partnership Advisory Board. Enhanced recovery from surgery in the UK: an audit of the Enhanced Recovery Partnership Programme 2009–2012. Br J Anaesth 2015. [Epub ahead of print].

FIVE KEY OPPORTUNITIES FOR VALUE IN THE PERIOPERATIVE JOURNEY

Perioperative medicine is in many ways a natural development of the ideas central to Enhanced Recovery after Surgery programs[25] with an added focus on the following:

i. Integration with care outside of the hospital before and after surgery
ii. Standardization of intraoperative care
iii. Effective use of in-hospital resources in the postoperative period

Five key opportunities for increasing value through perioperative medicine are highlighted.

Collaborative Decision Making

Collaborative (or shared) decision making puts the patient at the center of the surgical decision-making process.[26] The aim of this approach is to furnish patients and their carers with a comprehensive and readily understood picture of the harms and benefits of surgery, in order that they may make a well-informed decision grounded in the context of their own life. In general, this is likely to result in improved value: when decision aids are offered to people facing health treatment decisions they are more likely to lead to informed value-based decisions.[26] Specifically, in relation to discretionary surgery, the use of decision aids results in reduced rates of surgery without apparent adverse effects on health outcomes or satisfaction.[27] Such avoidance of unnecessary or ineffective surgery (where harm equals or exceeds benefit) benefits both the patient and the health care delivery system. However, achieving truly collaborative decision making may require pathway redesign before surgery to provide the patient with comprehensive information about likely benefits and harms at the same time. In the United Kingdom at present, it is common for potential benefits to be discussed in the context of the surgical consultation, although the full spectrum of harms may only be explored later during the anesthetic preassessment process, thus limiting the opportunity for patients to make a well-informed decision.

Lifestyle Modification Before Surgery

Exercise training (prehabilitation)[18] and smoking and alcohol cessation[19,20] offer opportunities to improve physiologic reserve and thereby reduce perioperative risk in the short time frame available between decision to operate and operation. Costs vary in this domain. Targeted in-hospital training programs are likely to have significant cost but may provide substantial outcome benefits. Smoking and alcohol cessation interventions are likely to be low cost but are unlikely to be effective in a substantial proportion of individuals. Long-term benefits contingent on sustained behavioral change, at least in a proportion of patients, may contribute substantial value for all these interventions, but measuring and correctly attributing these benefits are challenging.

Standardized In-Hospital Perioperative Care—Process Mapping and Improvement

Recent data support the notion that a proportion of the between-patient variation in delivered care and subsequent outcome is directly attributable to individual anesthesiologists (and institutions), rather than being explained by patient or surgical factors. Inter-anesthesiologist variations in practice are responsible for a proportion of observed process and outcome differences between patients. With respect to clinical outcomes, data from coronary artery bypass graft surgery in New York State show substantial adjusted mortality differences between different anesthesiologists.[28] With respect to process measures, the perioperative administration of fluids has been shown to be highly variable both between and within individual anesthesia providers, and provider identity was a stronger predictor of administered fluid volume than patient factors.[29] Such variability has been shown to be associated with variations in important outcomes, including cost and length of hospital stay.[30] Inter-insitutional differences in failure to rescue from complications following surgery are another example.[31] Such remarkable variation suggests substantial opportunity for improvement in patient outcomes and value, simply by reducing this unexplained provider-associated heterogeneity.

Achieving Full Recovery

Physical rehabilitation and exercise training, systematic review and optimization of the management of long-term conditions, identification and treatment of incident conditions, and targeted preventative medicine offer the possibility of improved long-term outcomes through the achievement of faster and more sustained recovery.[1] The optimal location, and therefore cost, of delivering such care is uncertain, but the long-term benefit in terms of improved duration and quality of life may be substantial.

Using Clinical Data for Quality Improvement

The effective use of clinical data is critical in the development of high-quality perioperative care and making best use of such data an important part of the role of the perioperative physician.[32] In the United Kingdom, national audit data have highlighted stark differences between institutions in quality of care and outcomes for specific patient groups, most notably those undergoing emergency procedures such as hip fracture and emergency laparotomy surgery.[33,34] Systematic audit and quality improvement may serve to level the playing field for patients undergoing diverse types of surgery. Routine effective feedback of quality indicators (clinical process and outcome data) can improve the quality of delivered care[35] and should be routine practice for anesthesiologists and perioperative physicians. Application of such an approach to emergency laparotomy surgery has been shown to reduce mortality.[36] Furthermore, collecting such data can also contribute to the development of increasingly sophisticated clinical risk and outcome measurement tools that can, in turn, facilitate the delivery of better collaborative decision making and the development of precision (individualized) medicine for this patient group.

FUTURE CONSIDERATIONS/SUMMARY

Value is delivered by perioperative medicine through the efficient practice of patient-centered, multidisciplinary, and integrated medical care of patients undergoing surgery (from the moment of contemplation of surgery until full recovery). Notwithstanding the complexity of defining value in health care, several specific opportunities arise to add value within the perioperative setting: collaborative decision making, lifestyle modification before surgery, standardization of in-hospital perioperative care, achieving full recovery after surgery, and the use of data for quality improvement. Perioperative medicine builds on the innovations of Enhanced Recovery after Surgery programs, and the success of such programs should provide reassurance that the journey toward perioperative medicine is likely to benefit patients and add value.

REFERENCES

1. Grocott MP, Pearse RM. Perioperative medicine. Br J Anaesth 2012;108(5): 723–6.

2. Cannesson M, Ani F, Mythen MM, et al. Anaesthesiology and perioperative medicine around the world: different names, same goals. Br J Anaesth 2015;114(1): 8–9.
3. Mythen MG, Berry C, Drake S, et al. Perioperative medicine: the pathway to better surgical care. London: Royal College of Anaesthetists; 2015.
4. Warner MA. The surgical home. ASA Newsl 2012;76(5):30–2.
5. Arrow K. Uncertainty and the welfare economics of medical care. Am Econ Rev 1963;53(5):941–73.
6. Smith A. An inquiry into the nature and causes of the wealth of nations. Oxford (United Kingdom): Oxford University Press; 1776 [1976].
7. Robbins LC. An essay on the nature and significance of economic science. London: Macmillan; 1932 [1935].
8. Appleby J. Spending on health and social care over the next 50 years. Why think long term? London: Kings Fund; 2013 [2013].
9. Congressional Budget Office. The long-term outlook for health care spending: sources of growth in projected federal spending on Medicare and Medicaid. Washington, DC: Congress of the United States Congressional Budget Office; 2007. Available at: www.cbo.gov/sites/default/files/cbofiles/ftpdocs/87xx/doc8758/11-13-lt-health.pdf. Accessed December 5, 2012.
10. Murphy KM, Topel RH. The value of health and longevity. J Polit Econ 2006; 114(5):871–904.
11. Buchanan J, Stubblebine WC. Externality. Economica 1962;29(116):371–84.
12. Available at: http://en.wikipedia.org/wiki/Value_(marketing). Accessed April 29, 2015.
13. Porter ME. What is value in health care? N Engl J Med 2010;363:2477–81.
14. Jolicoeur LM, Jones-Grizzle AJ, Boyer JG. Guidelines for performing a pharmacoeconomic analysis. Am J Hosp Pharm 1992;49(7):1741–7.
15. Wilkerson J. POCRI head vows not to do cost-effectiveness studies, but notes gray areas. 2011. InsideHealthPolicy.com. Accessed March 20, 2012.
16. McCabe C, Claxton K, Culyer AJ. The NICE cost-effectiveness threshold: what it is and what that means. Pharmacoeconomics 2008;26(9):733–44.
17. Black WC. The CE plane: a graphic representation of cost-effectiveness. Med Decis Making 1990;10(3):212–4.
18. Levett DZ, Grocott MP. Cardiopulmonary exercise testing, prehabilitation, and Enhanced Recovery after Surgery (ERAS). Can J Anaesth 2015;62(2): 131–42.
19. Thomsen T, Villebro N, Møller AM. Interventions for preoperative smoking cessation. Cochrane Database Syst Rev 2010;(7):CD002294.
20. Oppedal K, Møller AM, Pedersen B, et al. Preoperative alcohol cessation prior to elective surgery. Cochrane Database Syst Rev 2012;(7):CD008343.
21. Davis K, Stremikis K, Squires D, et al. Mirror, mirror on the wall: how the performance of the US health care system compares internationally, 2014 update. New York: The Commonwealth Fund; 2014.
22. Available at: http://www.nhs.uk/NHSEngland/thenhs/about/Pages/nhscoreprinciples.aspx. Accessed April 29, 2015.
23. Mythen MG. Spread and adoption of enhanced recovery from elective surgery in the English National Health Service. Can J Anaesth 2015;62(2):105–9.
24. Simpson JC, Moonesinghe SR, Grocott MP, et al, National Enhanced Recovery Partnership Advisory Board. Enhanced recovery from surgery in the UK: an audit of the enhanced recovery partnership programme 2009–2012. Br J Anaesth 2015. [Epub ahead of print].

25. Grocott MP, Martin DS, Mythen MG. Enhanced recovery pathways as a way to reduce surgical morbidity. Curr Opin Crit Care 2012;18(4):385–92.
26. Glance LG, Osler TM, Neuman MD. Redesigning surgical decision making for high-risk patients. N Engl J Med 2014;370(15):1379–81.
27. O'Connor AM, Bennett CL, Stacey D, et al. Decision aids for people facing health treatment or screening decisions. Cochrane Database Syst Rev 2009;(3):CD001431.
28. Glance LG, Kellermann AL, Hannan EL, et al. The impact of anesthesiologists on coronary artery bypass graft surgery outcomes. Anesth Analg 2015;120(3): 526–33.
29. Lilot M, Ehrenfeld JM, Lee C, et al. Variability in practice and factors predictive of total crystalloid administration during abdominal surgery: retrospective two-centre analysis. Br J Anaesth 2015;114(5):767–76.
30. Thacker C, Mythen M, et al, in press.
31. Ghaferi AA, Birkmeyer JD, Dimick JB. Variation in hospital mortality associated with inpatient surgery. N Engl J Med 2009;361:1368–75.
32. Grocott MP. Improving outcomes after surgery. BMJ 2009;339:b5173.
33. Saunders DI, Murray D, Pichel AC, et al, UK Emergency Laparotomy Network. Variations in mortality after emergency laparotomy: the first report of the UK Emergency Laparotomy Network. Br J Anaesth 2012;109(3):368–75.
34. White SM, Griffiths R, Holloway J, et al. Anaesthesia for proximal femoral fracture in the UK: first report from the NHS Hip Fracture Anaesthesia Network. Anaesthesia 2010;65(3):243–8.
35. Benn J, Arnold G, Wei I, et al. Using quality indicators in anaesthesia: feeding back data to improve care. Br J Anaesth 2012;109(1):80–91.
36. Huddart S, Peden CJ, Swart M, et al, ELPQuiC Collaborator Group. Use of a pathway quality improvement care bundle to reduce mortality after emergency laparotomy. Br J Surg 2015;102(1):57–66.

Demonstrating Value
A Case Study of Enhanced Recovery

Arvind Chandrakantan, MD, MBA[a], Tong Joo Gan, MD, MHS, FRCA[b],*

KEYWORDS

- ERAS • Protocol-driven care • Value-based care • Affordable Care Act
- Anesthetic approaches

KEY POINTS

- An enhanced recovery after surgery strategy will be increasingly adopted in the era of value-based care.
- The various elements in enhanced recovery protocols add value to the overall patient journey.
- Although the evidence varies considerably based on type of surgery and patient group, the team-based approach of care should be universally applied to patient care.

INTRODUCTION

Enhanced Recovery After Surgery (ERAS) is a multimodal perioperative care pathway designed to achieve early recovery for patients undergoing major surgery.[1] The basis of ERAS is promotion of best-practice guidelines across specialties to facilitate all aspects of the patient surgical journey. This process, by definition, involves coordination and integration of multiple medical specialties and nursing in order to ensure optimal outcomes. The available evidence for ERAS varies considerably. In colorectal surgery, which has the largest body of literature supporting ERAS, length of hospital stay has been shown to be reduced by as much as 30% and postoperative complications as much as 50%.[2]

Despite the improvement in outcomes and earlier discharge associated with ERAS, many hospital systems do not adhere to all aspects of the protocol.[3] A recent meta-analysis of the cost drivers suggests a strong benefit with ERAS protocols, despite

Funding sources: None.
Conflict of interest: None (A. Chandrakantan); research funding or honoraria from Acacia, Baxter, Edwards, Mallinckrodt, and Hospira (T.J. Gan).
[a] Department of Anesthesiology, Stony Brook Medicine, HSC Level 4, Room 060, Stony Brook, NY 11794-8480, USA; [b] Department of Anesthesiology, Stony Brook University School of Medicine, Stony Brook University, HSC Level 4, Room 060, Stony Brook, NY 11794-8480, USA
* Corresponding author.
E-mail address: tong.gan@stonybrookmedicine.edu

the limitation that indirect costs such as caregiver burden were not measured.[4] Despite the lack of data on uniform institutional control, there is a trend toward decreased length of stay (LOS) and decreased postoperative complications. This cost saving can be realized even in the implementation phase of ERAS protocols.[5]

However, the endgame in health care is patient outcome. Numerous studies involving multiple organ systems suggest a decreased LOS without a change in patient morbidity or mortality.[2,6] Another recent study also suggests that high-volume surgical centers with incipient protocols are associated with a lower rate of postoperative complications.[7] The study does not specify whether these centers use ERAS protocols, merely that high-volume centers are associated with lower postoperative complications.

WHAT IS VALUE?

Value in health care is defined as health care outcomes per dollar spent.[8] The nature of this equation is purely mathematical: either health care outcomes must be improved or the dollars spent per outcome must be reduced. The latter often leads to ill-conceived cost containment, because an initial period of spending can be recaptured by later savings.[9]

Reducing the Denominator in Value

Improving health care delivery is often a paradox in this context because money is required to realize the cost savings. However, in a recent model from an enhanced program at Duke University, cost savings were realized in 84.8% of iterations (**Fig. 1**).[10]

Value in the Context of the Affordable Care Act

The Affordable Care Act (ACA) has many provisions that affect physicians. Chief among these are the concept of bundled payments, as well as a focus on cost reduction.[11] The payments change the paradigm from being volume driven to value driven from the vantage point of the individual patient, as well as a default shift in that care becomes more integrative and collaborative rather than piecemeal. The impetus for the ACA was mainly driven by cost (the denominator of value), whereas the focus was mainly driven by the numerator (outcomes). Despite the United States spending the highest amount per capita on health care in the world, the outcomes were not better compared with other countries (**Fig. 2**).

Much of the drive also comes from countries that highly regulate cost, such as Japan. Although much of the cost can be attributed to insurance variability, which is essentially eliminated in a single payer system, there is also a pricing differential. Also complicating and expediting this discussion has been medical tourism, in which elective outpatient surgeries performed in developing countries are showing acceptable outcomes.[12] Although the subject is covered in detail later, the ACA accelerates the need for multidisciplinary coordination of care with the patient at the center, which is the crux of enhanced recovery.

How Is the Numerator Enhanced?

Improving health care outcomes is an often-quoted, widely misunderstood statement. Although, in the business world, value is measured over the long-term cycle of a given entity (eg, a stock), in the medical world, value is often measured and appropriately based on individual units. This system favored intervention rather than prevention until recently, and only the implementation of so-called never events seemed to signal an

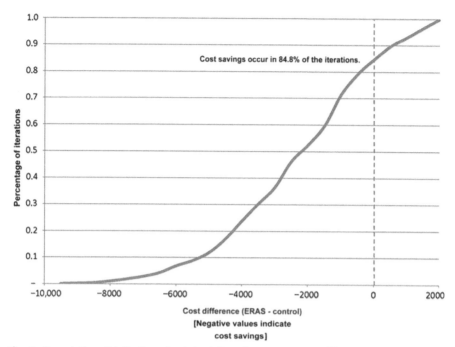

Fig. 1. Cumulative distribution chart depicting the percentage of bootstrap sample iterations in which the ERAS treatment strategy would be expected to be cost saving versus control using unadjusted values. (*From* Miller TE, Thacker JK, White WD, et al. Reduced length of hospital stay in colorectal surgery after implementation of an enhanced recovery protocol. Anesth Analg 2014;118:1058; with permission.)

emphasis away from individual processes. This phenomenon still exists, because each individual practitioner involved in the care of the patient still bills individually without necessarily being vested in the overall care delivered. However, with bundled payments being introduced, the model has to change because of the factors previously noted.

The definitions of outcomes in the context of health care are poorly defined. Does the outcome end at discharge? Thirty days after surgery without recurrence or readmission rate? There is often confusion among providers as to what the primary outcome should be for a given patient. Medicare and Medicaid seem to view the primary outcome in a 30-day context. For the purposes of this article, value is defined as decreasing direct cost, decreasing morbidity and/or mortality, and/or ensuring a more rapid transition toward the patient's preoperative state.

INTRODUCTION TO ENHANCED RECOVERY AFTER SURGERY PROTOCOLS

Although colon resection has become a fairly standardized and protocolized regimen, with an abundance of data supporting it, other regimens remain far less standardized. There have been several such regimens proposed, with varying levels of data supporting their value. The most widely cited remains colon resection (**Table 1**). Protocols on other procedures, for example, pancreaticoduodenectomy (**Table 2**), do not have as much evidence as colorectal resection.

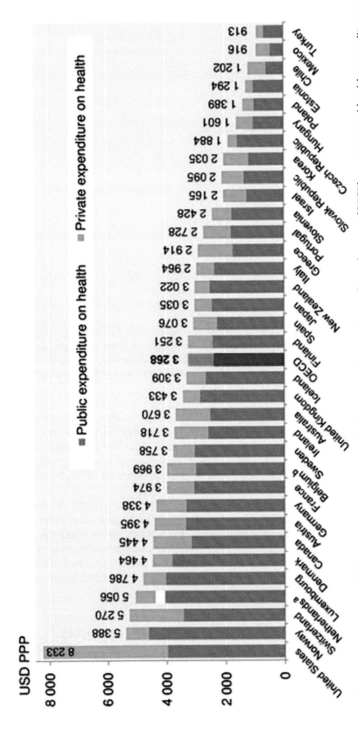

Fig. 2. The United States spends 2.5 times the Organisation for Economic Cooperation and Development (OECD) average: total health expenditure per capita, public and private 2010 (or nearest year). Information on data for Israel: http://dx.doi.org/10.1787/888932315602. aIn the Netherlands, it is not possible to clearly distinguish the public and private share related to investments. bTotal expenditure excluding investments. PPP, purchasing power parity. (*Data from* OECD Health Data 2012.)

Table 1
Guidelines for perioperative care in elective colonic surgery: ERAS Society recommendations

Item	Recommendation	Evidence Level	Recommendation Grade
Preoperative information, education, and counseling	Patients should routinely receive dedicated preoperative counseling	Low	Strong
Preoperative optimization	Preoperative medical optimization is necessary before surgery Smoking and alcohol consumption (alcohol abusers) should be stopped 4 wk before surgery	Alcohol: low Smoking: high	Strong
Preoperative bowel preparation	Mechanical bowel preparation should not be used routinely in colonic surgery	High	Strong
Preoperative fasting and carbohydrate treatment	Clear fluids should be allowed up to 2 h and solids up to 6 h before induction of anesthesia Preoperative oral carbohydrate treatment should be used routinely. In diabetic patients carbohydrate treatment can be given along with the diabetic medication	Solids and fluids: moderate Carbohydrate loading, overall: low Carbohydrate loading, diabetic patients: very low	Fasting guidelines: strong Preoperative carbohydrate drinks: strong Preoperative carbohydrate drinks, diabetic patients: weak
Preanesthetic medication	Patients should not routinely receive long-acting or short-acting sedative medication before surgery because it delays immediate postoperative recovery	High	Strong
Prophylaxis against thromboembolism	Patients should wear well-fitting compression stockings, have intermittent pneumatic compression, and receive pharmacologic prophylaxis with LMWH. Extended prophylaxis for 28 d should be given to patients with colorectal cancer	High	Strong
Antimicrobial prophylaxis and skin preparation	Routine prophylaxis using intravenous antibiotics should be given 30–60 min before initiating surgery Additional doses should be given during prolonged operations according to half-life of the drug used Preparation with chlorhexidine-alcohol should be used	High	Strong

(continued on next page)

Table 1
(continued)

Item	Recommendation	Evidence Level	Recommendation Grade
Standard anesthetic protocol	A standard anesthetic protocol allowing rapid awakening should be given The anesthetist should control fluid therapy, analgesia, and hemodynamic changes to reduce the metabolic stress response Open surgery: midthoracic epidural blocks using local anesthetics and low-dose opioids Laparoscopic surgery: spinal analgesia or morphine PCA is an alternative to epidural anesthesia	Rapid awakening: low Reduce stress response: moderate Open surgery: high Laparoscopic surgery: moderate	Strong
PONV	A multimodal approach to PONV prophylaxis should be adopted in all patients with ≥ 2 risk factors undergoing major colorectal surgery If PONV is present, treatment should be given using a multimodal approach	Low	Strong
Laparoscopy and modifications of surgical access	Laparoscopic surgery for colonic resections is recommended if the expertise is available	Oncology: high Morbidity: low Recovery/LOSH: moderate	Strong
Nasogastric intubation	Postoperative nasogastric tubes should not be used routinely Nasogastric tubes inserted during surgery should be removed before reversal of anesthesia	High	Strong
Preventing intraoperative hypothermia	Intraoperative maintenance of normothermia with a suitable warming device and warmed intravenous fluids should be used routinely to keep body temperature >36°C	High	Strong

Topic	Recommendation	Evidence level	Recommendation grade
Perioperative fluid management	Patients should receive intraoperative fluids (colloids and crystalloids) guided by flow measurements to optimize cardiac output Vasopressors should be considered for intraoperative and postoperative management of epidural-induced hypotension provided the patient is normovolemic The enteral route for fluid postoperatively should be used as early as possible, and intravenous fluids should be discontinued as soon as is practicable	Balanced crystalloids: high Flow measurement in open surgery: high Flow measurement in other patients: moderate Vasopressors: high Early enteral route: high	Strong
Drainage of peritoneal cavity after colonic anastomosis	Routine drainage is discouraged because it is an unsupported intervention that is likely to impair mobilization	High	Strong
Urinary drainage	Routine transurethral bladder drainage for 1–2 d is recommended The bladder catheter can be removed regardless of the usage or duration of thoracic epidural analgesia	Low	Routine bladder drainage: strong Early removal if epidural used: weak
Prevention of postoperative ileus	Midthoracic epidural analgesia and laparoscopic surgery should be used in colonic surgery if possible Fluid overload and nasogastric decompression should be avoided Chewing gum can be recommended, whereas oral magnesium and alvimopan may be included	Thoracic epidural, laparoscopy: high Chewing gum: moderate Oral magnesium, alvimopan: low	Thoracic epidural, fluid overload, nasogastric decompression, chewing gum, and alvimopan: strong Oral magnesium: weak

(continued on next page)

Table 1
(continued)

Item	Recommendation	Evidence Level	Recommendation Grade
Postoperative analgesia	Open surgery: TEA using low-dose local anesthetic and opioids. Laparoscopic surgery: an alternative to TEA is a carefully administered spinal analgesia with a low-dose, long-acting opioid	TEA, open surgery: high. Local anesthetic and opioid: moderate. TEA not mandatory in laparoscopic surgery: moderate	Strong
Perioperative nutritional care	Patients should be screened for nutritional status and, if at risk of undernutrition, given active nutritional support. Perioperative fasting should be minimized. Postoperatively patients should be encouraged to take normal food as soon as lucid after surgery. ONS may be used to supplement total intake	Postoperative early enteral feeding, safety: high. Improved recovery and reduction of morbidity: low. Perioperative ONS (well-fed patients): low. Perioperative ONS (malnourished patients): low. IN: low	Postoperative early feeding and perioperative ONS: strong. IN could be considered in open colonic resections: weak

Enhanced Recovery

637

Postoperative glucose control	Hyperglycemia is a risk factor for complications and should therefore be avoided Several interventions in the ERAS protocol affect insulin action/resistance, thereby improving glycemic control with no risk of causing hypoglycemia For ward-based patients, insulin should be used judiciously to maintain blood glucose as low as feasible with the available resources	Using stress-reducing elements of ERAS to minimize hyperglycemia: low Insulin treatment in the ICU: moderate Glycemic control in the ward setting: low	Using stress-reducing elements of ERAS to minimize hyperglycemia: strong Insulin treatment in the ICU (severe hyperglycemia): strong Insulin treatment in ICU (mild hyperglycemia): weak Insulin treatment in the ward setting: weak
Early mobilization	Prolonged immobilization increases the risk of pneumonia, insulin resistance, and muscle weakness. Patients should therefore be mobilized	Low	Strong

Abbreviations: ICU, intensive care unit; IN, immunonutrition; LMWH, low-molecular-weight heparin; LOSH, length of stay in hospital; ONS, oral nutritional supplements; PCA, patient-controlled anesthesia; PONV, postoperative nausea and vomiting; TEA, thoracic epidural anesthesia.

Table 2
Guidelines for perioperative care for pancreaticoduodenectomy: ERAS Society recommendations

Item	Summary and Recommendations	Evidence Level	Recommendation Grade
Preoperative counseling	Patients should receive dedicated preoperative counseling routinely	Low	Strong
Perioperative biliary drainage	Preoperative endoscopic biliary drainage should not be undertaken routinely in patients with a serum bilirubin concentration <250 µmol/L	Moderate	Weak
Preoperative smoking and alcohol consumption	For alcohol abusers, 1 mo of abstinence before surgery is beneficial and should be attempted. For daily smokers, 1 mo of abstinence before surgery is beneficial. For appropriate groups, both should be attempted	Alcohol abstention: low Smoking cessation: moderate	Strong
Preoperative nutrition	Routine use of preoperative artificial nutrition is not warranted, but significantly malnourished patients should be optimized with oral supplements or enteral nutrition preoperatively	Very low	Weak
Perioperative oral IN	The balance of evidence suggests that IN for 5–7 d perioperatively should be considered because it may reduce the rate of infectious complications in patients undergoing major open abdominal surgery	Moderate	Weak
Oral bowel preparation	Extrapolation of data from studies on colonic surgery and retrospective studies in PD show that MBP has no proven benefit. MBP should not be used	Moderate	Strong
Preoperative fasting and preoperative treatment with carbohydrates	Intake of clear fluids up to 2 h before anesthesia does not increase gastric residual volume and is recommended before elective surgery. Intake of solids should be withheld 6 h before anesthesia. Data extrapolation from studies in major surgery suggests that preoperative oral carbohydrate treatment should be given in patients without diabetes	Fluid intake: high Solid intake: low Carbohydrate loading: low	Fasting: strong Carbohydrate loading: strong
Preanesthetic medication	Data from studies on abdominal surgery show no evidence of clinical benefit from preoperative use of long-acting sedatives, and they should not be used routinely. Short-acting anxiolytics may be used for procedures such as insertion of epidural catheters	No long-acting sedatives: moderate	Weak

Intervention	Description	Evidence	Recommendation
Antithrombotic prophylaxis	LMWH reduces the risk of thromboembolic complications, and administration should be continued for 4 wk after hospital discharge. Concomitant use of epidural analgesia necessitates close adherence to safety guidelines. Mechanical measures should probably be added for patients at high risk	High	Strong
Antimicrobial prophylaxis and skin preparation	Antimicrobial prophylaxis prevents surgical-site infections, and should be used in a single-dose manner initiated 30–60 min before skin incision. Repeated intraoperative doses may be necessary depending on the half-life of the drug and duration of procedure	High	Strong
Epidural analgesia	Midthoracic epidurals are recommended based on data from studies on major open abdominal surgery showing superior pain relief and fewer respiratory complications compared with intravenous opioids	Pain: high Reduced respiratory complications: moderate Overall morbidity: low	Weak
Intravenous analgesia	Some evidence supports the use of PCA or intravenous lidocaine analgesic methods. There is insufficient information on outcome after PD	PCA: very low Intravenous lidocaine: moderate	Weak
Wound catheters and TAP block	Some evidence supports the use of wound catheters or TAP blocks in abdominal surgery. Results are conflicting and variable, and mostly from studies on lower gastrointestinal surgery	Wound catheters: moderate TAP blocks: moderate	Weak
PONV	Data from the literature on gastrointestinal surgery in patients at risk of PONV show the benefits of using different pharmacologic agents depending on the patient's PONV history, type of surgery, and type of anesthesia. Multimodal intervention during and after surgery is indicated	Low	Strong
Incision	The choice of incision is at the surgeon's discretion, and should be of a length sufficient to ensure good exposure	Very low	Strong
Avoiding hypothermia	Intraoperative hypothermia should be avoided by using cutaneous warming; ie, forced-air or circulating-water garment systems	High	Strong

(continued on next page)

Table 2
(continued)

Item	Summary and Recommendations	Evidence Level	Recommendation Grade
Postoperative glycemic control	Insulin resistance and hyperglycemia are strongly associated with postoperative morbidity and mortality. Treatment of hyperglycemia with intravenous insulin in the ICU setting improves outcomes but hypoglycemia remains a risk. Several ERAS protocol items attenuate insulin resistance and facilitate glycemic control without the risk of hypoglycemia. Hyperglycemia should be avoided as far as possible without introducing the risk of hypoglycemia	Low	Strong
Nasogastric intubation	Preemptive use of nasogastric tubes postoperatively does not improve outcomes, and their use is not warranted routinely	Moderate	Strong
Fluid balance	Near-zero fluid balance, avoiding overload of salt and water results in improved outcomes. Perioperative monitoring of stroke volume with transesophageal Doppler to optimize cardiac output with fluid boluses improves outcomes. Balanced crystalloids should be preferred to 0.9% saline	Fluid balance: high Esophageal Doppler: moderate Balanced crystalloids vs 0.9% saline: moderate	Strong
Perianastomotic drain	Early removal of drains after 72 h may be advisable in patients at low risk (ie, amylase content in drain <5000 U/L) for developing a pancreatic fistula. There is insufficient evidence to recommend routine use of drains, but their use is based only on low-level evidence	Early removal: high	Early removal: strong
Somatostatin analogues	Somatostatin and its analogues have no beneficial effects on outcome after PD. In general, their use is not warranted. Subgroup analyses for variability in the texture and duct size of the pancreas are not available	Moderate	Strong

Urinary drainage	Suprapubic catheterization is superior to transurethral catheterization if used for >4 d. Transurethral catheters can be removed safely on POD 1 or 2 unless otherwise indicated	High	For suprapubic: weak Transurethral catheter out POD 1–2: strong
DGE	There are no acknowledged strategies to avoid DGE. Artificial nutrition should be considered selectively in patients with DGE of long duration	Very low	Strong
Stimulation of bowel movement	A multimodal approach with epidural and near-zero fluid balance is recommended. Oral laxatives and chewing gum given postoperatively are safe, and may accelerate gastrointestinal transit	Laxatives: very low Chewing gum: low	Weak
Postoperative artificial nutrition	Patients should be allowed a normal diet after surgery without restrictions. They should be cautioned to begin carefully and increase intake according to tolerance over 3–4 d. Enteral tube feeding should be given only on specific indications and parenteral nutrition should not be used routinely	Early diet at will: moderate	Strong
Early and scheduled mobilization	Patients should be mobilized actively from the morning of the first POD and encouraged to meet daily targets for mobilization	Very low	Strong
Audit	Systematic improves compliance and clinical outcomes	Low	Strong

Abbreviations: DGE, delayed gastric emptying; IN, immunonutrition; MBP, mechanical bowel preparation; PD, pancreaticoduodenectomy; POD, postoperative day; TAP, transversus abdominis plane.

Although there is a clear argument for LOS reduction without a higher readmission rate, the components of the ERAS protocol that led to this reduction remain unclear.[13] It also remains unclear what the out-of-hospital burden is. Although this makes the cost metric easy to measure from the inpatient hospital stay point of view, it is difficult to measure from a patient-centric point of view. The cost benefit therefore seems proportional to the number of evidence-based interventions that can be strongly supported with data from a given ERAS protocol.[5]

Team Approach

One of the advantages of ERAS protocols is their team-based approach. It often requires multiple physicians and preoperative, intraoperative, and postoperative care providers, as well as nursing and other staff to be available and using the protocol. Numerous barriers have been identified in ERAS adoption,[14] including lack of institutional support or buy-in of other physicians. Up to 11% of physicians did not think that the evidence of ERAS was strong enough to support its adoption.[15] However, many surgeons pick and choose parts of the protocol that enhance the fast-track thinking in current practice.

The team-based approach in health care has been validated in multiple models all the way from intensive care unit[16] to primary care.[17] There have been improved patient outcomes in controlling index illnesses, as well as multiple end points with comorbid illnesses. There are also suggestions of greater patient satisfaction[16] but whether this by itself improves patient outcomes is poorly defined. There has been greater satisfaction by team members, which has been attributed to multiple factors.[18] Interdisciplinary collaboration also reduces readmission rates for reasons that are still to be elucidated.[19,20]

ELEMENTS OF THE ENHANCED RECOVERY AFTER SURGERY PROTOCOLS THAT HAVE BEEN SHOWN TO ENHANCE VALUE

There are multiple ERAS protocols available currently. Many are based on expert opinion or practice consensus in instances in which these recommendations cannot be formally tested because of risk of harm or futility. An excellent example is the use of routine preoperative nutrition optimization before gastrectomy[1] or preoperative medical optimization before any major surgery.

Surgical Approaches That Add or Subtract Value

Laparoscopic versus open

One of the well-documented interventions is the use of laparoscopic-assisted distal gastrectomy (LADG) in early gastric cancer. LADG has been proved to decrease time to oral intake, reduce intraoperative blood loss, shorten hospital stay, as well as reduce overall postoperative morbidity.[21–26] There are multiple studies documenting the advantages of the minimally invasive approach in bowel and pelvic surgery. These advantages include decreased LOS, decreased ileus, and faster transitions to oral intake.[27,28] Specific indications include benign disease[29,30] and colonic resections.[31,32]

Routine use of nasogastric or nasojejunal decompression

Routine use of nasogastric or nasojejunal decompression has not been shown to improve outcomes and hence is not recommended.[33–35] Their routine use increases the incidence of upper respiratory tract infections, gastroesophageal reflux, and postoperative vomiting.[35–38]

Routine use of perianastomotic drains
The routine use of perianastomotic postoperative drains has been shown to decrease value by increasing LOS as well as reoperation rates.[39,40]

Routine use of oral bowel preparation
In radical cystectomy surgery, as well as major abdominal surgery, oral bowel preparation can safely be omitted.[41,42] In elective colonic resection, which is the most studied of all ERAS protocols, preoperative mechanical bowel preparation is not recommended except in 2 instances: if intraoperative colonoscopy will be used to study an isolated lesion or if pelvic surgery is anticipated with a proximal diversion. In the former case, there is fear of being unable to localize the lesion; in the latter there is a trend toward harm without bowel preparation, which has not been conclusively proved.[43,44]

Urinary bladder catheterization
The high incidence of nosocomial urinary tract infections, and associated morbidity and cost, makes this one of the focal points of ERAS protocols. One of the complicating factors behind the timing of catheter removal involves retention caused by epidural catheter placement. The literature suggests removing urinary catheters, if feasible, within the first postoperative day, even if the epidural catheter is to be left in place.[45]

Gum chewing
A surprisingly low-cost, low-risk adjuvant that has shown early return in bowel function is mastication with chewing gum immediately following surgery.[46,47] There has been demonstrable benefit in reduction of LOS and decrease in systemic inflammatory makers.[48] This benefit seems to be tempered in patients in whom an aggressive early enteral regimen is pursued.[49]

Other therapies
Although many measures seem intuitive, there are some data to support these practices, including early oral feeding after major surgery and early ambulation.[50] Although not easily quantifiable, patient team dynamics are essential in the implementation of an ERAS program and add value to the patient's outcome.

ANESTHETIC APPROACHES THAT ADD VALUE
Low-molecular-weight Heparin

The use of low-molecular-weight heparin (LMWH) to prevent venous thromboembolism has been proved to be of value in a variety of studies for multiple procedures.[51–54] The timing of LMWH has to be balanced with placement and removal of epidural catheters.[55]

Nil by Mouth After Midnight

There is currently a shift from the generic nil by mouth after midnight to a more patient-friendly approach, which recommends carbohydrate loading just before surgery. Reductions in hunger, length of stay, and anxiety, as well as decreased postoperative insulin resistance, have been shown.[56–58] This effect has been shown to change the LOS by up to 1 day.[59] There are also the intangibles that add to the value of care, including preservation of skeletal muscle mass, and more positive nitrogen balance (as a function of muscle catabolism during surgery suggesting decreased stress response).[53,60–64] In addition, many of the postoperative indicators that add to cost, including postoperative nausea and vomiting, have been shown to be decreased by the use of carbohydrate loading.[65] More recently, these conclusions have been challenged, with several studies showing minimal benefit in LOS.[59,66,67] These studies showed that preoperative carbohydrate loading was safe in the preoperative setting.

Prophylactic Antibiotic Use

The use of prophylactic antibiotics has been shown to be of value in colorectal surgery in the prevention of infectious complications.[68] Efficacy has been validated for preoperative oral antibiotics[69] as well as the combination of intravenous and oral antibiotics.[70] Oral antibiotic use should be started preoperatively and extend into the postoperative period.

Pain Management

Epidural analgesia has immediate benefits in pain control and averting the undesirable consequences of parenteral opioids. Some of the benefits include improved pulmonary function, especially following abdominal surgery; decreased ileus; and early ambulation.[71–75] Their benefit can vary significantly, with proven benefit in colorectal surgery to mildly positive or equivocal benefit in other surgical cohorts. Many of these studies had small numbers of patients. The colorectal surgery data also show value for spinal anesthetics.[76] Opioid and benzodiazepine use in the elderly can also lead to postoperative cognitive dysfunction, and therefore opioid-sparing techniques are desirable in this cohort of patients.[77]

The utility of multimodal analgesia has been shown in numerous studies across the spectrum of surgical procedures.[78] Use of this technique improves pain scores, results in greater patient satisfaction, decreases LOS, and decreases the incidence of chronic pain. The approach is highly recommended in an ERAS protocol. Multimodal analgesia is not limited to intravenous and neuraxial anesthetics. Surgery-specific regional anesthesia, including transversus abdominis plane (TAP) catheters, has been implemented successfully within ERAS protocols and showed improvement in outcomes.[79] Adjuvant nonpharmacologic therapies, such as acupuncture, music therapy, and hypnosis, have been implemented with mixed results; however, at least 1 study recommends them because of minimal risk.[80]

Postoperative Nausea and Vomiting

Postoperative nausea and/or emesis often delays patient discharge and results in significant discomfort.[81] The use of a multimodal prophylactic antiemetic approach has been shown to optimize both the outcome and the cost for patients.[82]

Euthermia

Euthermia has also been shown to be of benefit in both the ambulatory and inpatient settings. Management of thermal status optimizes intraoperative outcomes (transfusion requirements) as well as postoperative outcomes (LOS, postoperative recovery, wound infections).[83–88] The consequences of failure to manage thermal status vary from minor responses, such as shivering, to major sequelae, including major myocardial events.[89] In the authors' institution, a preoperative warming device is offered to all patients at the ambulatory center to facilitate early discharge. This practice has been well established as an effective means of preventing intraoperative hypothermia.[90]

Fluid Administration

Excessive fluid administration has also been shown to increase complication rates and lead to delayed discharge.[91–95] Although avoiding overhydration seems to be the goal, there is a crucial lack of data in patients in ASA (American Society of

Anesthesiologists) class 3 or greater. Therefore, most experts in fluid management suggest individually tailored fluid therapy in these patients, using appropriate hemodynamic monitors when needed, including but not limited to arterial lines, esophageal Doppler, and central venous catheters. Fluid regulation versus vasopressor therapy to maintain mean arterial pressure is of particular importance in intra-abdominal surgery, in which the lack of splanchnic autoregulation makes these patients more dependent on mean arterial pressure and cardiac output.[96]

The practice of augmenting stroke volume or cardiac output by optimizing fluid management is known as goal-directed fluid therapy. A recent meta-analysis validated the use of goal-directed fluid therapy rather than the traditional fluid management approach.[97] There was no benefit to the using colloids rather than crystalloids for goal-directed therapy.[98] There are data that indicate that goal-directed therapy also seems to benefit all patients; however, morbidity and mortality benefits are well shown in high-risk subgroups.[99] More recent data also advocate a goal of zero balance as well as permissive oliguria in the management of fluid in the perioperative period.[100]

SUMMARY

An ERAS strategy will be increasingly adopted in the era of value-based care. The various elements in each ERAS protocol are likely to add value to the overall patient surgical journey. Although the evidence varies considerably based on the type of surgery and patient group, the team-based approach of care should be universally applied to patient care.

REFERENCES

1. Mortensen K, Nilsson M, Slim K, et al. Consensus guidelines for enhanced recovery after gastrectomy: enhanced recovery after surgery (ERAS®) society recommendations. Br J Surg 2014;101:1209–29.
2. Varadhan KK, Neal KR, Dejong CH, et al. The enhanced recovery after surgery (ERAS) pathway for patients undergoing major elective open colorectal surgery: a meta-analysis of randomized controlled trials. Clin Nutr 2010;29:434–40.
3. Ahmed J, Khan S, Lim M, et al. Enhanced recovery after surgery protocols - compliance and variations in practice during routine colorectal surgery. Colorectal Dis 2012;14:1045–51.
4. Lee L, Li C, Landry T, et al. A systematic review of economic evaluations of enhanced recovery pathways for colorectal surgery. Ann Surg 2014;259:670–6.
5. Roulin D, Donadini A, Gander S, et al. Cost-effectiveness of the implementation of an enhanced recovery protocol for colorectal surgery. Br J Surg 2013;100: 1108–14.
6. Coolsen MM, van Dam RM, van der Wilt AA, et al. Systematic review and meta-analysis of enhanced recovery after pancreatic surgery with particular emphasis on pancreaticoduodenectomies. World J Surg 2013;37:1909–18.
7. Tsai TC, Joynt KE, Orav EJ, et al. Variation in surgical-readmission rates and quality of hospital care. N Engl J Med 2013;369:1134–42.
8. Porter ME, Teisberg EO. Redefining competition in health care. Harv Bus Rev 2004;82:64–76, 136.
9. Relph S, Bell A, Sivashanmugarajan V, et al. Cost effectiveness of enhanced recovery after surgery programme for vaginal hysterectomy: a comparison of pre and post-implementation expenditures. Int J Health Plann Manage 2014;29: 399–406.

10. Miller TE, Thacker JK, White WD, et al. Reduced length of hospital stay in colorectal surgery after implementation of an enhanced recovery protocol. Anesth Analg 2014;118:1052–61.
11. Forum on Medical and Public Health Preparedness for Catastrophic Events; Board on Health Sciences Policy; Board on Health Care Services; Institute of Medicine: National Academies Press, 2014.
12. Maulik P. Service quality and patient's satisfaction in medical tourism with special reference to Gujarat state. Ex J Int Multidisc Man St 2013;3:33–8. Available at: http://www.indianjournals.com/ijor.aspx?target=ijor:xijmms&volume=3&issue=1&article=004.
13. Nussbaum DP, Penne K, Stinnett SS, et al. A standardized care plan is associated with shorter hospital length of stay in patients undergoing pancreaticoduodenectomy. J Surg Res 2015;193:237–45.
14. Kahokehr A, Sammour T, Zargar-Shoshtari K, et al. Implementation of ERAS and how to overcome the barriers. Int J Surg 2009;7:16–9.
15. Kahokehr A, Robertson P, Sammour T, et al. Perioperative care: a survey of New Zealand and Australian colorectal surgeons. Colorectal Dis 2011;13:1308–13.
16. Kim MM, Barnato AE, Angus DC, et al. The effect of multidisciplinary care teams on intensive care unit mortality. Arch Intern Med 2010;170:369–76.
17. Katon WJ, Lin EH, Von Korff M, et al. Collaborative care for patients with depression and chronic illnesses. N Engl J Med 2010;363:2611–20.
18. Youngwerth J, Twaddle M. Cultures of interdisciplinary teams: how to foster good dynamics. J Palliat Med 2011;14:650–4.
19. Propp KM, Apker J, Zabava Ford WS, et al. Meeting the complex needs of the health care team: identification of nurse-team communication practices perceived to enhance patient outcomes. Qual Health Res 2010;20:15–28.
20. Partnership for Health in Aging Workgroup on Interdisciplinary Team Training in Geriatrics. Position statement on interdisciplinary team training in geriatrics: an essential component of quality health care for older adults. J Am Geriatr Soc 2014;62:961–5.
21. Ding J, Liao GQ, Liu HL, et al. Meta-analysis of laparoscopy-assisted distal gastrectomy with D2 lymph node dissection for gastric cancer. J Surg Oncol 2012;105:297–303.
22. Memon MA, Khan S, Yunus RM, et al. Meta-analysis of laparoscopic and open distal gastrectomy for gastric carcinoma. Surg Endosc 2008;22:1781–9.
23. Ohtani H, Tamamori Y, Noguchi K, et al. A meta-analysis of randomized controlled trials that compared laparoscopy-assisted and open distal gastrectomy for early gastric cancer. J Gastrointest Surg 2010;14:958–64.
24. Vinuela EF, Gonen M, Brennan MF, et al. Laparoscopic versus open distal gastrectomy for gastric cancer: a meta-analysis of randomized controlled trials and high-quality nonrandomized studies. Ann Surg 2012;255:446–56.
25. Yakoub D, Athanasiou T, Tekkis P, et al. Laparoscopic assisted distal gastrectomy for early gastric cancer: is it an alternative to the open approach? Surg Oncol 2009;18:322–33.
26. Zeng YK, Yang ZL, Peng JS, et al. Laparoscopy-assisted versus open distal gastrectomy for early gastric cancer: evidence from randomized and nonrandomized clinical trials. Ann Surg 2012;256:39–52.
27. Doorly MG, Senagore AJ. Pathogenesis and clinical and economic consequences of postoperative ileus. Surg Clin North Am 2012;92:259–72, viii.

28. Kang CY, Chaudhry OO, Halabi WJ, et al. Outcomes of laparoscopic colorectal surgery: data from the nationwide inpatient sample 2009. Am J Surg 2012;204: 952–7.
29. Fajardo AD, Dharmarajan S, George V, et al. Laparoscopic versus open 2-stage ileal pouch: laparoscopic approach allows for faster restoration of intestinal continuity. J Am Coll Surg 2010;211:377–83.
30. Wu XJ, He XS, Zhou XY, et al. The role of laparoscopic surgery for ulcerative colitis: systematic review with meta-analysis. Int J Colorectal Dis 2010;25:949–57.
31. Wang G, Jiang ZW, Zhao K, et al. Fast track rehabilitation programme enhances functional recovery after laparoscopic colonic resection. Hepatogastroenterology 2012;59:2158–63.
32. Vlug MS, Wind J, Hollmann MW, et al. Laparoscopy in combination with fast track multimodal management is the best perioperative strategy in patients undergoing colonic surgery: a randomized clinical trial (LAFA-study). Ann Surg 2011;254:868–75.
33. Chen K, Mou YP, Xu XW, et al. Necessity of routine nasogastric decompression after gastrectomy for gastric cancer: a meta-analysis. Zhonghua Yi Xue Za Zhi 2012;92:1841–4 [in Chinese].
34. Yang Z, Zheng Q, Wang Z. Meta-analysis of the need for nasogastric or nasojejunal decompression after gastrectomy for gastric cancer. Br J Surg 2008; 95:809–16.
35. Nelson R, Edwards S, Tse B. Prophylactic nasogastric decompression after abdominal surgery. Cochrane Database Syst Rev 2007;(3):CD004929.
36. Manning BJ, Winter DC, McGreal G, et al. Nasogastric intubation causes gastroesophageal reflux in patients undergoing elective laparotomy. Surgery 2001; 130:788–91.
37. Rao W, Zhang X, Zhang J, et al. The role of nasogastric tube in decompression after elective colon and rectum surgery: a meta-analysis. Int J Colorectal Dis 2011;26:423–9.
38. Jottard K, Hoff C, Maessen J, et al. Life and death of the nasogastric tube in elective colonic surgery in the Netherlands. Clin Nutr 2009;28:26–8.
39. Kumar M, Yang SB, Jaiswal VK, et al. Is prophylactic placement of drains necessary after subtotal gastrectomy? World J Gastroenterol 2007;13:3738–41.
40. Kim J, Lee J, Hyung WJ, et al. Gastric cancer surgery without drains: a prospective randomized trial. J Gastrointest Surg 2004;8:727–32.
41. Tabibi A, Simforoosh N, Basiri A, et al. Bowel preparation versus no preparation before ileal urinary diversion. Urology 2007;70:654–8.
42. Xu R, Zhao X, Zhong Z, et al. No advantage is gained by preoperative bowel preparation in radical cystectomy and ileal conduit: a randomized controlled trial of 86 patients. Int Urol Nephrol 2010;42:947–50.
43. Guenaga KF, Matos D, Wille-Jorgensen P. Mechanical bowel preparation for elective colorectal surgery. Cochrane Database Syst Rev 2011;(9):CD001544.
44. Bretagnol F, Panis Y, Rullier E, et al. Rectal cancer surgery with or without bowel preparation: the French GRECCAR III multicenter single-blinded randomized trial. Ann Surg 2010;252:863–8.
45. Tripepi-Bova KA, Sun Z, Mason D, et al. Early removal of urinary catheters in patients with thoracic epidural catheters. J Nurs Care Qual 2013;28:340–4.
46. Fitzgerald JE, Ahmed I. Systematic review and meta-analysis of chewing-gum therapy in the reduction of postoperative paralytic ileus following gastrointestinal surgery. World J Surg 2009;33:2557–66.

47. Ho YM, Smith SR, Pockney P, et al. A meta-analysis on the effect of sham feeding following colectomy: should gum chewing be included in enhanced recovery after surgery protocols? Dis Colon Rectum 2014;57:115–26.
48. van den Heijkant TC, Costes LM, van der Lee DG, et al. Randomized clinical trial of the effect of gum chewing on postoperative ileus and inflammation in colorectal surgery. Br J Surg 2015;102:202–11.
49. Zaghiyan K, Felder S, Ovsepyan G, et al. A prospective randomized controlled trial of sugared chewing gum on gastrointestinal recovery after major colorectal surgery in patients managed with early enteral feeding. Dis Colon Rectum 2013; 56:328–35.
50. Yang D, He W, Zhang S, et al. Fast-track surgery improves postoperative clinical recovery and immunity after elective surgery for colorectal carcinoma: randomized controlled clinical trial. World J Surg 2012;36:1874–80.
51. Koch A, Bouges S, Ziegler S, et al. Low molecular weight heparin and unfractionated heparin in thrombosis prophylaxis after major surgical intervention: update of previous meta-analyses. Br J Surg 1997;84:750–9.
52. Rasmussen MS, Jorgensen LN, Wille-Jorgensen P. Prolonged thromboprophylaxis with low molecular weight heparin for abdominal or pelvic surgery. Cochrane Database Syst Rev 2009;(1):CD004318.
53. Nygren J, Thacker J, Carli F, et al. Guidelines for perioperative care in elective rectal/pelvic surgery: enhanced recovery after surgery (ERAS®) society recommendations. World J Surg 2013;37:285–305.
54. Hill J, Treasure T. Reducing the risk of venous thromboembolism (deep vein thrombosis and pulmonary embolism) in patients admitted to hospital: summary of the NICE guideline. Heart 2010;96:879–82.
55. O'Rourke MR, Rosenquist RW. Applying the ASRA guidelines to the use of low-molecular-weight heparin thromboprophylaxis in major orthopedic surgery. J Arthroplasty 2004;19:919–22.
56. Hausel J, Nygren J, Lagerkranser M, et al. A carbohydrate-rich drink reduces preoperative discomfort in elective surgery patients. Anesth Analg 2001;93: 1344–50.
57. Helminen H, Viitanen H, Sajanti J. Effect of preoperative intravenous carbohydrate loading on preoperative discomfort in elective surgery patients. Eur J Anaesthesiol 2009;26:123–7.
58. Brady M, Kinn S, Ness V, et al. Preoperative fasting for preventing perioperative complications in children. Cochrane Database Syst Rev 2009;(4): CD005285.
59. Awad S, Varadhan KK, Ljungqvist O, et al. A meta-analysis of randomised controlled trials on preoperative oral carbohydrate treatment in elective surgery. Clin Nutr 2013;32:34–44.
60. Nygren J. The metabolic effects of fasting and surgery. Best Pract Res Clin Anaesthesiol 2006;20:429–38.
61. Crowe PJ, Dennison A, Royle GT. The effect of pre-operative glucose loading on postoperative nitrogen metabolism. Br J Surg 1984;71:635–7.
62. Svanfeldt M, Thorell A, Hausel J, et al. Randomized clinical trial of the effect of preoperative oral carbohydrate treatment on postoperative whole-body protein and glucose kinetics. Br J Surg 2007;94:1342–50.
63. Yuill KA, Richardson RA, Davidson HI, et al. The administration of an oral carbohydrate-containing fluid prior to major elective upper-gastrointestinal surgery preserves skeletal muscle mass postoperatively–a randomised clinical trial. Clin Nutr 2005;24:32–7.

64. Henriksen MG, Hessov I, Dela F, et al. Effects of preoperative oral carbohydrates and peptides on postoperative endocrine response, mobilization, nutrition and muscle function in abdominal surgery. Acta Anaesthesiol Scand 2003;47:191–9.

65. Gustafsson UO, Hausel J, Thorell A, et al. Adherence to the enhanced recovery after surgery protocol and outcomes after colorectal cancer surgery. Arch Surg 2011;146:571–7.

66. Smith MD, McCall J, Plank L, et al. Preoperative carbohydrate treatment for enhancing recovery after elective surgery. Cochrane Database Syst Rev 2014;(8):CD009161.

67. Webster J, Osborne SR, Gill R, et al. Does preoperative oral carbohydrate reduce hospital stay? A randomized trial. AORN J 2014;99:233–42.

68. Nelson RL, Gladman E, Barbateskovic M. Antimicrobial prophylaxis for colorectal surgery. Cochrane Database Syst Rev 2014;(5):CD001181.

69. Cannon JA, Altom LK, Deierhoi RJ, et al. Preoperative oral antibiotics reduce surgical site infection following elective colorectal resections. Dis Colon Rectum 2012;55:1160–6.

70. Bellows CF, Mills KT, Kelly TN, et al. Combination of oral non-absorbable and intravenous antibiotics versus intravenous antibiotics alone in the prevention of surgical site infections after colorectal surgery: a meta-analysis of randomized controlled trials. Tech Coloproctol 2011;15:385–95.

71. Block BM, Liu SS, Rowlingson AJ, et al. Efficacy of postoperative epidural analgesia: a meta-analysis. JAMA 2003;290:2455–63.

72. Werawatganon T, Charuluxanun S. Patient controlled intravenous opioid analgesia versus continuous epidural analgesia for pain after intra-abdominal surgery. Cochrane Database Syst Rev 2005;(1):CD004088.

73. Jorgensen H, Wetterslev J, Moiniche S, et al. Epidural local anaesthetics versus opioid-based analgesic regimens on postoperative gastrointestinal paralysis, PONV and pain after abdominal surgery. Cochrane Database Syst Rev 2000;(4):CD001893.

74. Popping DM, Elia N, Marret E, et al. Protective effects of epidural analgesia on pulmonary complications after abdominal and thoracic surgery: a meta-analysis. Arch Surg 2008;143:990–9 [discussion: 1000].

75. Zhu Z, Wang C, Xu C, et al. Influence of patient-controlled epidural analgesia versus patient-controlled intravenous analgesia on postoperative pain control and recovery after gastrectomy for gastric cancer: a prospective randomized trial. Gastric Cancer 2013;16:193–200.

76. Levy BF, Scott MJ, Fawcett W, et al. Randomized clinical trial of epidural, spinal or patient-controlled analgesia for patients undergoing laparoscopic colorectal surgery. Br J Surg 2011;98:1068–78.

77. Krenk L, Rasmussen LS, Kehlet H. New insights into the pathophysiology of postoperative cognitive dysfunction. Acta Anaesthesiol Scand 2010;54:951–6.

78. Chandrakantan A, Glass PS. Multimodal therapies for postoperative nausea and vomiting, and pain. Br J Anaesth 2011;107(Suppl 1):i27–40.

79. Favuzza J, Delaney CP. Outcomes of discharge after elective laparoscopic colorectal surgery with transversus abdominis plane blocks and enhanced recovery pathway. J Am Coll Surg 2013;217:503–6.

80. Tan M, Law LS, Gan TJ. Optimizing pain management to facilitate enhanced recovery after surgery pathways. Can J Anaesth 2015;62:203–18.

81. Smith H, Smith EJ. Postoperative nausea and vomiting. Ann Palliat Med 2012;1:94–102.

82. Apfel CC, Korttila K, Abdalla M, et al. A factorial trial of six interventions for the prevention of postoperative nausea and vomiting. N Engl J Med 2004;350:2441–51.

83. Kurz A, Sessler DI, Lenhardt R. Perioperative normothermia to reduce the incidence of surgical-wound infection and shorten hospitalization. Study of Wound Infection and Temperature Group. N Engl J Med 1996;334:1209–15.

84. Scott EM, Buckland R. A systematic review of intraoperative warming to prevent postoperative complications. AORN J 2006;83:1090–104, 1107–13.

85. Frank SM, Fleisher LA, Breslow MJ, et al. Perioperative maintenance of normothermia reduces the incidence of morbid cardiac events. A randomized clinical trial. JAMA 1997;277:1127–34.

86. Rajagopalan S, Mascha E, Na J, et al. The effects of mild perioperative hypothermia on blood loss and transfusion requirement. Anesthesiology 2008;108: 71–7.

87. Lenhardt R, Marker E, Goll V, et al. Mild intraoperative hypothermia prolongs postanesthetic recovery. Anesthesiology 1997;87:1318–23.

88. Wong PF, Kumar S, Bohra A, et al. Randomized clinical trial of perioperative systemic warming in major elective abdominal surgery. Br J Surg 2007;94:421–6.

89. Sessler D. Temperature monitoring: the consequences and prevention of mild perioperative hypothermia. S Afr J Anes Analg 2014;20:25–31. Available at: http://www.tandfonline.com/doi/pdf/10.1080/22201173.2014.10844560.

90. Pu Y, Cen G, Sun J, et al. Warming with an underbody warming system reduces intraoperative hypothermia in patients undergoing laparoscopic gastrointestinal surgery: a randomized controlled study. Int J Nurs Stud 2014;51:181–9.

91. Brandstrup B, Tonnesen H, Beier-Holgersen R, et al. Effects of intravenous fluid restriction on postoperative complications: comparison of two perioperative fluid regimens: a randomized assessor-blinded multicenter trial. Ann Surg 2003;238: 641–8.

92. Chowdhury AH, Lobo DN. Fluids and gastrointestinal function. Curr Opin Clin Nutr Metab Care 2011;14:469–76.

93. Lobo DN, Bostock KA, Neal KR, et al. Effect of salt and water balance on recovery of gastrointestinal function after elective colonic resection: a randomised controlled trial. Lancet 2002;359:1812–8.

94. Lobo DN. Fluid overload and surgical outcome: another piece in the jigsaw. Ann Surg 2009;249:186–8.

95. Varadhan KK, Lobo DN. A meta-analysis of randomised controlled trials of intravenous fluid therapy in major elective open abdominal surgery: getting the balance right. Proc Nutr Soc 2010;69:488–98.

96. Correa TD, Vuda M, Takala J, et al. Increasing mean arterial blood pressure in sepsis: effects on fluid balance, vasopressor load and renal function. Crit Care 2013;17:R21.

97. Corcoran T, Rhodes JE, Clarke S, et al. Perioperative fluid management strategies in major surgery: a stratified meta-analysis. Anesth Analg 2012;114: 640–51.

98. Yates DR, Davies SJ, Milner HE, et al. Crystalloid or colloid for goal-directed fluid therapy in colorectal surgery. Br J Anaesth 2014;112:281–9.

99. Cecconi M, Corredor C, Arulkumaran N, et al. Clinical review: goal-directed therapy-what is the evidence in surgical patients? The effect on different risk groups. Crit Care 2013;17:209.

100. Miller TE, Roche AM, Mythen M. Fluid management and goal-directed therapy as an adjunct to enhanced recovery after surgery (ERAS). Can J Anaesth 2015;62:158–68.

Value from the Patients' and Payers' Perspectives

Joshua H. Atkins, MD, PhD[a], Lee A. Fleisher, MD, FACC, FAHA[b],*

KEYWORDS

- Value • Quality • Cost • Perioperative • Patient-reported outcome measures
- Perspective • Patient

KEY POINTS

- Value incorporates both quality and costs.
- The value components incorporated in the determination of quality and costs depend on the perspective taken, for example, payer and patient.
- Although major morbidity and mortality are important determinants of quality, the patient perspective must include return to baseline function and quality of life.

The costs of health care continue to increase in the United States and most of the industrialized world. Despite the increasing costs of care, the outcomes achieved have remained unchanged for decades. Michael Porter and colleagues[1] propose that the overarching strategy for health care should be to improve value for patients, whereby value is defined as patient outcomes achieved in relation to the amount of money spent. Further, they think that "only through achieving better outcomes that matter to patients, reducing the costs required to deliver those outcomes, or both can medicine unite the interests of all key stakeholders."

Value within the paradigm of anesthetic care is difficult to separate from that of the entire perioperative experience. The US federal government has developed the value-based payment plan that began as bonuses on physician reporting of specific metrics to more recently imposing penalties for not reporting. The Centers for Medicare and Medicaid Services (CMS) also incorporated these measures into hospital-based payments, and most hospitals incorporated these metrics as part of their contracts with physicians. The initial focus by both the CMS and the American Society of Anesthesiologists for anesthesiologist metrics was process measures, evidence-based processes of care that are linked to outcomes. These initial metrics included some

[a] Department of Anesthesiology and Critical Care, Perelman School of Medicine of the University of Pennsylvania, Philadelphia, PA 19104, USA; [b] Perelman School of Medicine of the University of Pennsylvania, Philadelphia, PA 19104, USA
* Corresponding author. University of Pennsylvania, 3400 Spruce Street Dulles 680, Philadelphia, PA 19104.
E-mail address: lee.fleisher@Uphs.upenn.edu

Anesthesiology Clin 33 (2015) 651–658
http://dx.doi.org/10.1016/j.anclin.2015.07.001   anesthesiology.theclinics.com
1932-2275/15/$ – see front matter © 2015 Elsevier Inc. All rights reserved.

of the Surgical Care Improvement Project measures, such as antibiotic timing within 1 hour of incision and choice of antibiotic for surgery. These measures were also incorporated into private plans like Blue Cross/Blue Shield with physicians and hospitals.

The other major change in the payment area has been the move to bundled care. Although slow to be adopted, Sylvia Burwell,[2] Secretary of Health and Human Services, has recently written that the federal government's plan is to accelerate the movement to alternative payment models, including bundled payments, over the next 3 years. Bundled care involves paying a single amount to hospitals that includes the payments for both hospital and physician care. It frequently also incorporates payment for care for a time frame after hospital discharge that can vary from 30 days to 90 days. The premise of such a payment approach is that the hospitals will take responsibility for delivering the highest quality care for the lowest total cost (ie, value). Although the Accountable Care Organization model linking provider payments to quality and outcomes has recently demonstrated national cost savings,[3] the barriers to implementation of bundled payments may be substantial.[4] This article focuses on the value equation from the perspective of the payer and patients.

VALUE FROM THE PAYERS' PERSPECTIVE

Currently, the method to judge the outcome side of the value equation is complex and varies according the group using the data. Death is an easily assessed outcome, and risk-adjusted mortality can be measured and used in the value equation. Risk-adjusted complication rates can also be used by the payers to assess value; however, complications increase costs and must be incorporated into the cost side of the equation as a function of resource utilization. Furthermore, each surgical procedure or medical treatment would require a defined set of outcomes, which require risk adjustment. For example, risk-adjusted outcomes have been well defined in the Society of Thoracic Surgeons (STS); but this has required decades of research and a great deal of resources to collect in their database.[5] Defining similar risk-adjusted outcomes across the broad spectrum of surgery and interventional procedures would be a substantial undertaking. Other surgical specialty groups, including anesthesiologists, have or are developing databases to demonstrate value. These databases include the National Anesthesia Core Outcome Registry established by the American Society of Anesthesiologists National Quality Institute and the Multicenter Perioperative Outcomes Group established by Kevin Tremper and the University of Michigan.[6,7]

In the United States, there is a burgeoning growth of quality metrics that can be used on the quality side of the equation. These quality metrics can be defined by the specialty itself, such as the STS risk-adjusted mortality and complications, or by the payers, such as private insurers or Medicare. Initially many of the measures were oriented around process, but there is increasing pressure to focus on outcomes. In order to truly measure quality of care for patients, even from the payers' perspective, quality metrics must be focused on outcomes.

Patrick Conway[8], the chief medical officer of the CMS, has articulated the following goals of performance measurement (**Table 1**).[9]

- Meaningful quality measures increasingly need to transition away from setting-specific, narrow snapshots.
- Reorient and align measures around patient-centered outcomes that span across settings.
- Measures need to be based on patient-centered episodes of care.
- Capture measurement at 3 main levels (ie, individual clinician, group/facility, population/community).

Table 1
Recommendations for improving health care measurement

Group	Recommendations
Clinicians	Develop and implement measures relevant to your practice; explore data to find opportunities for improving care; and build the necessary data-collection infrastructure (eg, registries).
Patients and consumers	Call for transparent quality measurement and reporting, and participate in efforts to collect patient-reported outcome information.
Payers	Align with other payers on a smaller required set of high-impact and outcome-oriented measures.
Employers and purchasers	Purchase health care by meaningful, actionable quality and cost measures, focused on outcomes and team- and system-level performance.

Adapted from Cassel CK, Conway PH, Delbanco SF, et al. Getting more performance from performance measurement. N Engl J Med 2014;371:2146; with permission.

When discussing value from the payers' perspective, we must acknowledge that they may be different between public (governmental) payers and private insurers or self-insured companies. For example, outcomes may include return to work if the insurer is closely aligned or is the actual employer. If the insurer pays separately for postdischarge care, this may also be important to assess with regard to value. Because value incorporates quality and costs, each must be examined separately. With the move toward bundles of care, Medicare and other insurers have shifted costs to the provider; therefore, assessing value of postdischarge care and the costs of that care has become more important to the provider. If care is delivered under a traditional fee-for-service model, the individual components of care may actually be reimbursed separately; therefore, optimizing patients' experience and care may not be achieved.

Payers, especially Medicare, have also focused on readmissions as a measure of quality. Readmissions are costly but are also important outcomes for patients, providers, and payers. However, they may not measure the primary concern for patients, which may be better reflected by disability-free days at home. The assessment of an episode of hospital care has now been extended outside the hospital through the inclusion of bundles. The length of any bundle, such as 30, 60, or 90 days after the initial treatment, can drive the providers to a greater extent to modify care but should improve care in a patient-centered manner. As the value perspective is further developed over the next several years, the quality side of the equation will need to become better defined.

As anesthesiologists, we tend to focus on value from the perspective of achieving good outcomes after surgery. We have frequently focused on morbidity and mortality directly attributable to anesthesia care. However, the payers' perspective would include the outcomes of the entire team. Shared accountability with our surgical colleagues and the hospital for the entire episode of care is critical to our success. The other articles in this issue clearly articulate the means of anesthesiologists becoming more involved in the patients' care.

Value from the perspective of pain management is all about achieving a return to baseline function as quickly as possible and at the lowest cost. There are numerous scales that can be used to assess functional status in chronic pain. One perspective may simply be return to work for working individuals. This outcome is clearly important to patients and should be a focus for anesthesiologists who perform chronic pain management. Another manner in which anesthesiologists could add value is the time to diagnosis. The quicker individuals can be diagnosed and treated for their problems, the more value they can offer. This point is extremely important in the area of back pain. For example, getting the correct diagnosis and initiating treatment quickly may have a benefit on both symptoms and costs, for example, being the gatekeeper for chronic medication management, epidural injections, and laminectomy.

Costs are also impacted by the perspective and coverage decisions of the payers. Both Medicare and private insurers are incorporating value-based purchasing into their reimbursement schemes.[10,11] As noted earlier, the schema for bundles of care shifts the postdischarge costs to the providers and the rate set for the bundle includes a certain rate of complications and admissions. As improved and more coordinated care is achieved, these costs will continue to decrease and there will be increasing pressure to decrease reimbursement further. Outside of bundled care, the actual coverage may impact the total calculation of costs because some of the costs may be covered, whereas others may be assumed by the providers (physicians, hospitals, home health, long-term acute care, and so forth) and patients.[12,13]

VALUE FROM THE PATIENTS' PERSPECTIVE

Value to patients may include overall clinical outcome, total out-of-pocket costs, or quicker return to productive or revenue-generating activities. With respect to the outcomes side of the equation, clearly mortality and major morbidity are a primary focus for patients. However, with respect to the surgical arena, it is important to return back to baseline function or improve functioning if that is the goal of the surgical intervention. Traditionally, anesthesiologists have focused on anesthesia- related outcomes, such as pain and nausea and vomiting. However, there is increasing emphasis on the concept of shared accountability measures in which traditionally surgical recovery is shared with the anesthesia team. With the development of enhanced recovery after surgery protocols, it is becoming clear that anesthesiologists can help influence this recovery.[14,15]

Joint responsibility with their surgical colleagues at the Royal College of Surgeons is a hallmark of the program in England. The Perioperative Surgical Home attempts to put the anesthesiologist at the center of this pathway, although many institutions are developing joint programs with their surgical colleagues.[16] Therefore, a much broader definition of value to patients must be the focus, particularly for more invasive or larger surgical procedures. Even for outpatient surgery, a focus on returning patients to baseline function should be a goal.

Shulman and colleagues[17] in Australia have begun to use the World Health Organization Disability Activity Scale (WHODAS) as a means of measuring the outcome that he thinks is most important to patients: the speed at which they recover from disability after surgery. If overall days at home during any time are of high value to patients, a single readmission, when able to restore overall function quicker or for longer, may not be as relevant to patients from the cost perspective as a slower recovery of function through less intensive outpatient care. Future focus will clearly include these important new, broader measures and perspectives in identifying the value of the anesthesiologist.

From the patients' perspective, cost of care includes those costs that patients directly pay for a particular episode of care. This cost can include payment to the hospital or physicians for the uninsured or required copayments. It can also include copayments for medications and total pharmaceutical costs for uncovered medications. The costs also include lost wages for patients and lost wages for other care providers. Given the short length of stay for many surgical procedures, spouses, children, or parents may be required to be caregivers even after the initial procedure or hospitalization. Any copayments for home health or skilled nursing facilities or rehabilitation should also be considered. Therefore, value to patients should consider all of these costs, and any reduction in patient-related costs should be perceived and calculated as increasing the value.

A SPECIFIC EXAMPLE

Obstructive sleep apnea (OSA) is an important example of how anesthesiologists fulfill the value equation for patients and payers. OSA is a major population health problem with high prevalence and increasing incidence that may affect as many as 19 million adults in the United States (Harvard Medical School Division of Sleep Medicine/McKinsey & Co Price of Fatigue https://www.google.com/?gws_rd=ssl#q=price+of+fatigue). OSA is associated with significant direct and indirect health care costs.[18] From the employers' and payers' perspectives, untreated OSA is associated with substantial reduction in worker productivity, higher incidence of disability, and increased health care utilization.[19–22] Despite this, most patients with OSA are undiagnosed. Untreated OSA is associated with more severe systemic disease, including hypertension and heart failure[23]; OSA represents an increasingly prominent signal in perioperative litigation records.[24,25]

The American Academy of Sleep Medicine recently reported 3 quality measures of focus for OSA: improved detection, improved quality of life, and decreased cardiovascular risk through treatment.[24] Anesthesiologists are positioned to impact each of these measures and have a direct impact on general long-term outcomes and perioperative risk; longer-term morbidity; and accelerated return to productive, preoperative baseline. We engage OSA patients from a systems vantage point being knowledgeable of the physiologic implications of OSA, the complexity of perioperative management, and the potential complications associated with the combination of OSA, surgery, sedation, and opioid therapy (**Box 1**).

Patients with undiagnosed or poorly managed OSA frequently present for interventional procedures. The anesthesia preoperative assessment often presents the first opportunity for OSA diagnosis to be formally considered and directly discussed with patients.[26] The bedside STOP-BANG questionnaire is a validated tool developed by anesthesiologists with high sensitivity to determine the likelihood of mild, moderate, or severe sleep apnea.[27] A high score on the anesthesia perioperative screen may trigger differential perioperative management and monitoring with the potential to reduce immediate risk or perioperative adverse events.[28] A positive screen will also lead to referral for outpatient workup and treatment with impact on future costs of care for the payers and patients' quality of life. Anesthesiologists will play a central role in the prescribing of postprocedure continuous positive airway pressure (CPAP) for in-patient surgical procedures and for determining suitability of discharge for outpatients.

Although CPAP remains the gold standard therapy, overall patient compliance with prescribed therapy is low and the lack of alternative options can be frustrating for patients and lead to depression and decreased productivity.[29] The anesthesia preoperative interview can identify nonadherence with recommended CPAP and can trigger conversations with both patients and primary physicians about barriers to use and alternative therapies, such as surgery, to improve care. A variety of surgical procedures have been developed to treat OSA. These procedures are not without morbidity such that patients and procedures must be carefully selected. Accurate

---

Box 1
Spectrum of anesthesiologist role in the care of patients with OSA

Preoperative

Screening (eg, STOP-BANG)

Risk counseling (perioperative and beyond)

Referral for sleep study and sleep-related cardiovascular assessment

Identification of CPAP nonadherence

Development of multidisciplinary care pathways

Intraoperative

Expert airway management

CPAP-BiPAP during procedural sedation

Anesthetic drug selection

Regional and multimodal analgesia

Drug-induced sleep endoscopy

Postoperative

Develop postoperative monitoring protocols: PACU, wards

Prescribe postoperative CPAP/BiPAP and level of care

Plan analgesic regimen (postoperative and hospitalized, nonoperative patients with acute and chronic pain)

Discharge planning

Trial and implement new respiratory monitoring technologies

Abbreviations: BiPAP, bilevel positive airway pressure; CPAP, continuous positive airway pressure; PACU, postanesthesia care unit.

---

determination of the sites of obstruction is not straightforward, and multiple areas are often implicated. Drug-induced sleep endoscopy (DISE) is a technique pioneered in England to assess the airway by nasopharyngoscopy under the effects of sedative hypnotics.[30] Anesthesiologists have been central in the clinical development of anesthetic approaches to sedative-hypnotic dosing. New approaches to propofol dosing for DISE have demonstrated high reliability to achieve obstruction in a short period of time with adequate safety.[31] DISE has previously been restricted to centers with niche experts in sleep apnea. Development of generalizable, high-fidelity anesthetic approaches to DISE should improve access to this important diagnostic tool. There is growing evidence that the results of DISE impact and alter surgical planning.[32] DISE can also be used to both titrate and assess the efficacy of CPAP. DISE may reduce the need for 2-night in-house sleep studies that are both resource intensive and unpalatable for patients. Availability of appropriately experienced anesthesiologists and ear, nose, and throat surgeons to incorporate DISE into diagnostic pathways may reduce the likelihood and associated costs of failed surgery while at the same time promoting appropriate, effective treatment of patients who would otherwise go untreated.

Opioid medications put all patients at significant risk of sleep-disordered breathing with both acute perioperative and chronic use.[32] Although inadequate pain control is a significant source of patient dissatisfaction, opioids, benzodiazepines, and hypnotics alter sleep architecture. Patients with OSA may be particularly vulnerable to the effects of opioids on respiratory control centers and be at an increased risk of central sleep apnea with associated adverse events. With experience in acute and chronic pain, anesthesiologists provide critical expertise to guide opioid and multimodal analgesic therapy for patients with sleep apnea in the perioperative and medical settings. Similarly, anesthesiologists have substantial experience with the use of novel respiratory monitors during general anesthesia and sedation.[33] This expertise can be extended to guide the appropriate selection and application of new respiratory monitoring technologies on the inpatient ward and in remote monitoring capacity for risk reduction and quality improvement in the perioperative period. It will be important to build these value contributions into care bundles and develop shared outcome measures for value-cost models across the spectrum of care for patients with OSA.

REFERENCES

1. Porter ME, Pabo EA, Lee TH. Redesigning primary care: a strategic vision to improve value by organizing around patients' needs. Health Aff (Millwood) 2013;32(3):516–25.
2. Burwell SM. Setting value-based payment goals–HHS efforts to improve U.S. health care. N Engl J Med 2015;372:897–9.
3. Rajkumar R, Press MJ, Conway PH. The CMS innovation center–a five-year self-assessment. N Engl J Med 2015;372:1981–3.
4. Ridgely MS, de Vries D, Bozic KJ, et al. Bundled payment fails to gain a foothold in California: the experience of the IHA bundled payment demonstration. Health Aff (Millwood) 2014;33:1345–52.
5. Shahian DM, Jacobs JP, Edwards FH, et al. The Society of Thoracic Surgeons national database. Heart 2013;99:1494–501.
6. Dutton RP. The National Anesthesia Clinical Outcomes Registry: a sustainable model for the information age? EGEMS (Wash DC) 2014;2:1070.
7. Tremper KK. Anesthesiology: from patient safety to population outcomes: the 49th annual Rovenstine lecture. Anesthesiology 2011;114:755–70.
8. Conway PH, Mostashari F, Clancy C. The Future of Quality Measurement for Improvement and Accountability. JAMA 2013;309(21):2215–6.
9. Cassel CK, Conway PH, Delbanco SF, et al. Getting more performance from performance measurement. N Engl J Med 2014;371:2145–7.
10. Conrad D, Grembowski D, Gibbons C, et al. A report on eight early-stage state and regional projects testing value-based payment. Health Aff (Millwood) 2013; 32:998–1006.
11. Sprague L. Seeking value in Medicare: performance measurement for clinical professionals. Issue Brief Natl Health Policy Forum 2013;(852):1–11.
12. Bernard DM, Johansson P, Fang Z. Out-of-pocket healthcare expenditure burdens among nonelderly adults with hypertension. Am J Manag Care 2014;20: 406–13.
13. Scott AR, Rush AJ 3rd, Naik AD, et al. Surgical follow-up costs disproportionately impact low-income patients. J Surg Res 2015. [Epub ahead of print].
14. Feldman LS, Lee L, Fiore J Jr. What outcomes are important in the assessment of enhanced recovery after surgery (ERAS) pathways? Can J Anaesth 2015;62: 120–30.
15. McLeod RS, Aarts MA, Chung F, et al. Development of an enhanced recovery after surgery guideline and implementation strategy based on the knowledge-to-action cycle. Ann Surg 2015. [Epub ahead of print].

16. Kain ZN, Hwang J, Warner MA. Disruptive innovation and the specialty of anesthesiology: the case for the perioperative surgical home. Anesth Analg 2015;120:1155–7.
17. Shulman MA, Myles PS, Chan MT, et al. Measurement of disability-free survival after surgery. Anesthesiology 2015;122:524–36.
18. Tarasiuk A, Reuveni H. The economic impact of obstructive sleep apnea. Curr Opin Pulm Med 2013;19:639–44.
19. Bahammam A, Delaive K, Ronald J, et al. Health care utilization in males with obstructive sleep apnea syndrome two years after diagnosis and treatment. Sleep 1999;22:740–7.
20. Banno K, Ramsey C, Walld R, et al. Expenditure on health care in obese women with and without sleep apnea. Sleep 2009;32:247–52.
21. Diaz K, Faverio P, Hospenthal A, et al. Obstructive sleep apnea is associated with higher healthcare utilization in elderly patients. Ann Thorac Med 2014;9:92–8.
22. Hirsch Allen AJ, Bansback N, Ayas NT. The effect of OSA on work disability and work-related injuries. Chest 2015;147:1422–8.
23. Floras JS. Hypertension and sleep apnea. Can J Cardiol 2015;31:889–97.
24. Fouladpour N, Jesudoss R, Bolden N, et al. Perioperative complications in obstructive sleep apnea patients undergoing surgery: a review of the legal literature. Anesth Analg 2015. [Epub ahead of print].
25. Tolisano AM, Bager JM. Sleep surgery and medical malpractice. Laryngoscope 2014;124:E250–4.
26. Hofer J, Chung E, Sweitzer BJ. Preanesthesia evaluation for ambulatory surgery: do we make a difference? Curr Opin Anaesthesiol 2013;26:669–76.
27. Chung F, Subramanyam R, Liao P, et al. High STOP-Bang score indicates a high probability of obstructive sleep apnoea. Br J Anaesth 2012;108:768–75.
28. Seet E, Chung F. Management of sleep apnea in adults - functional algorithms for the perioperative period: continuing professional development. Can J Anaesth 2010;57:849–64.
29. Mokhlesi B, Guralnick AS. CPAP adherence during the perioperative period. J Clin Sleep Med 2013;9:733–4.
30. Croft CB, Pringle M. Sleep nasendoscopy: a technique of assessment in snoring and obstructive sleep apnoea. Clin Otolaryngol Allied Sci 1991;16:504–9.
31. Atkins JH, Mandel JE, Rosanova G. Safety and efficacy of drug-induced sleep endoscopy using a probability ramp propofol infusion system in patients with severe obstructive sleep apnea. Anesth Analg 2014;119:805–10.
32. Eichler C, Sommer JU, Stuck BA, et al. Does drug-induced sleep endoscopy change the treatment concept of patients with snoring and obstructive sleep apnea? Sleep Breath 2013;17:63–8.
33. Atkins JH, Mandel JE. Performance of Masimo rainbow acoustic monitoring for tracking changing respiratory rates under laryngeal mask airway general anesthesia for surgical procedures in the operating room: a prospective observational study. Anesth Analg 2014;119:1307–14.

"What Have We Done for Us Lately?" – Defining Performance and Value at the Individual Clinician Level

 CrossMark

Katherine H. Dobie, MD[a], Vikram Tiwari, MBA, PhD[b],
Warren S. Sandberg, MD, PhD[c],*

KEYWORDS

- Clinical productivity measurement • Private practice • Academic practice
- Perioperative surgical home • Operating room management • Medical direction
- Compensation • Career development

KEY POINTS

- Consolidation in anesthesiology practice and throughout the rest of health care creates pressure to improve the product offered by anesthesia professionals.
- Anesthesia professionals must offer more than a reliable stream of anesthetized, operated, and recovered patients to remain competitive.
- By pooling resources and application of leadership effort, large departments and group practices can conduct individual-level value assessments of clinicians, using, for example, balanced scorecard approaches.
- Individual clinicians can be incentivized to improve their personal value proposition by rewards, such as compensation plans tied to desired outcomes.
- By creating an interlocking program of ongoing assessment, career development coaching and opportunities, and compensation, departments and group practices can return value to individual clinicians by curating and accelerating their career and capability development.

Disclosures: None of the authors has any conflicts of interest to disclose.
[a] Division of Ambulatory Anesthesiology, Department of Anesthesiology, Vanderbilt University School of Medicine, 1211 21st Avenue South, MAB722, Nashville, TN 37212, USA;
[b] Department of Anesthesiology, Vanderbilt University Hospital, Vanderbilt University School of Medicine, 1211 21st Avenue South, MAB722, Nashville, TN 37212, USA; [c] Department of Anesthesiology, Vanderbilt University School of Medicine, 1211 21st Avenue South, MAB722, Nashville, TN 37212, USA
* Corresponding author.
E-mail address: warren.sandberg@vanderbilt.edu

INTRODUCTION

The individual value of an anesthesiologist can be defined as the quotient of output (broadly conceived) over cost. Individual value is thus measured by assessing traditional (and nontraditional) outputs and the cost, driven by compensation plus overhead. What are the costs, products, and changes in product offering that influence the value of an individual anesthesiologist? This focused review touches on the cost of anesthesia care but mostly focuses on value-adding activities and a discussion of how anesthesia groups can use compensation to recognize and incentivize effort that improves anesthesiologists' economic value to the health system.

Cost of Anesthesiologists and the Economic Climate of 2015

The direct cost of anesthesiology services is driven almost entirely by personnel salaries and to some extent by the decisions anesthesiologists make that influence personnel costs elsewhere (there are also harder to quantify indirect costs, such as those arising from poor anesthesiology decisions that then have a negative impact on long-term patient outcomes downstream from the anesthetic event).[1] As of 2009, the cost beyond collections of an academic anesthesiologist, in terms of the support required to finance an academic anesthesia department, was $111,000 per clinical faculty member after accounting for hospital support for certified registered nurse anesthetists (CRNAs).[2] The fully loaded cost for 278 days (weekdays plus weekend call) of anesthesia coverage, including reasonable call, vacation (and vacation coverage), and fringe benefits, seems to remain at approximately $600,000 per year, whether in private (Sandberg WS, personal communication from chief of a midsized Midwestern private practice group, 2015) or academic practice.[2] Perhaps somewhat prematurely, the authors speculated in 2009 that anesthesiology services were under sufficient pricing pressure to allow a disruptive innovation to begin to replace the traditional provider-in-room model.[3] Only recently has one example of such technology (the Sedasys system [Ethicon, Cincinnati, OH, USA]) gained Food and Drug Administration approval for use in gastrointestinal procedures requiring moderate sedation, but the authors maintain that the writing is on the proverbial wall for one-person-one-patient anesthesia care. Meanwhile, the Affordable Care Act and the Great Recession have come to pass. The health care spending curve has been bent, and payers (ultimately US employers) are allowing smaller increases in US health care spending than previously. Nevertheless, the salary cost of an academic anesthesiologist has continued to rise at the rate of approximately 1% per year – lower than the rate of inflation but still costing more than can be supported by direct revenue alone.[4]

Anesthesiology, like the rest of the health care industry, is in the midst of a mergers-and-acquisitions frenzy. There are multiple objectives driving mergers and acquisitions in anesthesiology: economies of scale with respect to practice management, revenue cycle, and benefits, as well as the potential for more control over clinician performance, pricing power with payers, gaining control of salary costs, and better negotiating position with hospitals over support stipends to cover otherwise uncompensated work, such as medical direction, call, or quality improvement. At the same time, anesthesiologists are attempting to redefine themselves, and thereby their value, as perioperative physicians – agents of the perioperative surgical home. Their performance in this new role is important to hospitals, because perioperative environments and immediate postsurgical care account for a large percentage of hospital expenditures and revenues. More and more, hospitals expect anesthesiologists to drive efficiencies, patient experience, throughput, and innovation of care for the surgical home.[5] Putting aside patients for the moment, the economic goal of health care is to make money for shareholders and owners by creating headroom between the cost of practice and net revenue. This will call upon anesthesiologists to successfully demonstrate a value that directly influences revenue and cost-saving within the surgical home environment, independent of revenue generated by their own fee-for-service work.

How do anesthesiologists respond? Academic and private practice groups alike are facing strong economic pressures to justify their costs (almost entirely salary/income costs) and are accommodating real reductions in spending on their services.[6] In the cost of service discussion, anesthesiologist costs and CRNA costs are on the same order of magnitude, so are considered parts of a whole in this analysis; anesthesiologists and CRNAs are in the same boat together. For the rest of this exposition, all anesthesia professionals are considered one group, despite current political conflicts between professional societies.

As consolidation advances, private practice as previously known (solo to 50-physician group partnerships) is endangered – consolidating into large regional groups, practice management groups, and hospital-employed groups – all comprising 50 to 1000 providers. This trend reduces academic practices to relatively small entities, albeit with the additional overhead of education and research that private practice usually does not bear. The consequence of this consolidation of private practices into larger groups is that private and academic practice look more similar in terms of scope, size, and expectations for real participation in perioperative system leadership, systems, and quality improvement and innovation than ever before. Consequently, the definitions and discussion of the value of an individual clinician to the parent organization become broadly generalizable across settings. In other words, thousands of anesthesiologists in the United States are now employed by groups of 100 or more practitioners. If individual clinicians want to avoid becoming numbers (think: "Inspected by #43" sticker on the base of a big box store table lamp), they will want to work in systems that value factors beyond most clinical productivity for lowest unit cost. All this is to say that the exposition of how individual clinician value in anesthesiology is assessed applies to CRNAs and physician anesthesiologists, in academic and private practice alike.

Increasing Value by Taking on New Roles

In a time when physicians are under more scrutiny to define value added than ever before, anesthesiologists have failed to fully understand (or, at least, to articulate) their contribution to the value equation as it relates to the bottom line for a hospital – specifically, the total perioperative package, including the surgical home. Conversely, perhaps facilities have failed to recognize that although they may pay stipends to gap fund anesthesiologists' costs for non–revenue-generating work, the savings and profit that the anesthesiologists contribute to the their bottom lines may exceed estimates and far exceed the stipends. In other words, perhaps anesthesiologists have yet to clearly articulate to their clients and stakeholders the anesthesiologists' true contribution to the value equation. If that is true, then 2 important questions are raised that will determine the vitality and trajectory of tomorrow's anesthesiologists: who will define their value, and how will they do it?

What is the anesthesiologist's product? Levitt, in 1980,[7] introduced the concept of the product as a multilevel construct, with core attributes and key differentiators that serve to distinguish it from competitors' offerings. **Fig. 1** illustrates this concept, in a general sense, after Levitt, in the left panel, and with a sketch analogy to the anesthesiologist's product, in the right panel. The literature is filled with examples of anesthesiologist value beyond the safely anesthetized and recovered patient; articles in the literature include instances of perioperative analytics,[8–12] operating room (OR) and perioperative system redesign,[13–20] OR management,[1,21] clinical informatics driving

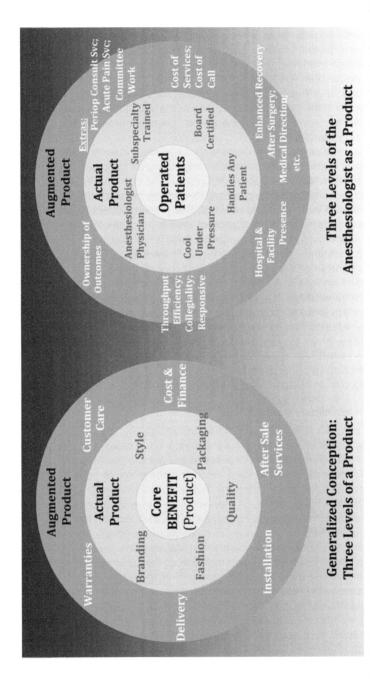

Fig. 1. Levels of a product. The 3 levels of a product mapped onto anesthesiology. Anesthesiologists have typically attended to the first and second levels of product importance. Scrupulous attention to improving the appeal of the third level – the Augmented Product – is necessary to secure a future for anesthesiologists. (*Adapted from* Levitt T. Marketing success through differentiation - of anything. Harvard Business Review. Graduate School of Business Administration, Harvard University; 1980. p. 83–91.)

revenue and outcomes improvements,[22–27] safety initiatives,[28] and nascent surgical home projects.[17,29] With a few exceptions, what is missing from the literature is how to translate that value into real dollars and where it fits into the value equation that the host institution can use to determine or justify salary support to cover anesthesiology activities that support their mission but do not generate American Society of Anesthesiologists (ASA) unit revenue.

Traditionally, anesthesiologists have been obligate system-level physicians, dependent on costly, highly regulated physical locations (ORs, procedure rooms, and intensive care units) as the venue to do their revenue-generating work. With the advent of the surgical home, anesthesiologists are rediscovering the perioperative physician and broadening their practice environments beyond the traditional OR, procedural venues, and ICU. The success of this rapidly evolving concept will be critically important to the economic landscape of surgical health care's future. Anesthesiologists can incorporate the perioperative home into their value proposition by demonstrating cost savings – or, said another way, revenue generation through the same skills and attitudes they bring to efficient OR management.[21,29] They can achieve this by making more capacity in surgical beds by reducing hospital length of stay (LOS), by squeezing more patients safely through the ORs at ambulatory surgery centers (ASCs), by innovating and educating, and by collaborative operational leadership in the surgical home.

Many academic programs across the country are piloting perioperative services and are beginning to demonstrate decreased surgical LOS through their stewardship.[30] Similarly, medical directors of high-quality, high-throughput ASCs are excellent examples of the perioperative physician at work, successfully facilitating the tenets of the surgical home (coordination, resource optimization, and personalization) for ambulatory patients.[5] An ASC's medical director adds value through clinical innovation and systems improvement so that the ASC can take on more complexity while minimizing bad outcomes, with fewer resources, more efficiently (operational leadership) and safely, all the while opening up surgical beds (whether directly in the ASC to increase real-time throughput or indirectly by moving cases from the hospital to the ASC). But this is not all an anesthesiologist can bring to the host institution, particularly in academics, where most faculty are expected to contribute in nonclinical ways (education and research). Perhaps it is time to consider these contributions specifically as they relate to the hospital's bottom line. For example, one way to look at education and research is that each provides a tremendous value for institutional sales and marketing, with respect to contracting and in attracting patients. Moreover, a well-aligned academic faculty, when focused on education, clinical effectiveness, research, and quality improvement science, improves the capabilities of the host institution.

As economic pressures continue to exert stress on the health care system, hospitals and academic institutions will be aggressively re-evaluating all the terms in the value equation; this will inherently put the burden on anesthesiologists (and other physicians) to re-evaluate and redefine themselves to respond in a way that aligns their mission to their host institutions more closely than ever. Said another way, the onus will be on the anesthesiologist to define and message the perioperative physician/leader/educator/scholar's role in the surgical home that translates to real economic benefits for their host institutions. The articles comprising the rest of this issue treat a range of approaches to increasing anesthesiologist value through new product offerings, including OR management, cost management, lean principles, and extras, such as enhanced recovery after surgery and the perioperative surgical home (see **Fig. 1**). The remainder of this article brings the value assessment home to the individual clinician, with a focus on how compensation is used as an incentive to continually improve the value proposition of an anesthesia group to its host institution.

INDIVIDUAL-LEVEL VALUE ASSESSMENT

As the definitions of group-level and individual-level value of anesthesiologists-as-product rapidly evolve, performance assessment tools and compensation plans must closely follow suit to proactively facilitate (motivate) the growth and development of the future anesthesiologist.

Performance Assessment: a Balanced Scorecard

An anesthesiology group assesses its members' contribution to patient care and their value to the overall department and patient population in a variety of ways. Measuring value begs an outputs/inputs framework, where the inputs are primarily clinician salary, and the outputs have traditionally been the number of safely operated patients and the resulting ASA units. As described previously and in other articles in this issue, outputs have dramatically expanded to include meaningful engagement in operational and clinical effectiveness improvement efforts as well as system-level quality and patient experience improvement work. This, in turn, demands a value assessment beyond how many ASA units the clinician generates per day.

Recognizing the multiple avenues for contribution to mission in a large anesthesia group, a balanced scorecard approach is used to assess provider value in the Vanderbilt Department of Anesthesiology (**Box 1**). Rewards are assigned for value via a

---

Box 1
Balanced scorecard major elements (not all areas apply to all faculty)

ASA units and wRVUs produced

Academic accomplishments[a]

Resident evaluations[b,43]

Attendance at departmental leadership, management, and educational meetings

Quality process measure scores

Ongoing professional practice evaluations, indicating clinician is in group[c]

Demonstrated effectiveness in designated leadership roles

Minimal or no yellow/red flags (see **Box 2**)

[a] The department operates a detailed academic achievement award system, with a focus on durable academic products and educational efforts. Recognition is given for all educational work, spanning the continuum from undergraduate students to attending physicians. Learning formats that can be archived and publically accessed are preferentially valued, as are externally facing educational activities that bring recognition to the home department. The program also recognizes external funding for research. Publication in all forms is recognized. The highest value is assigned to work that advances knowledge (broadly defined) in medicine and appears in high-impact, peer-reviewed journals.
[b] The department considers scores and written comments. Comments are most highly weighted. Department favorably views comments about how well the faculty challenge the learner to improve and about the quality of faculty-to-trainee feedback. Resident feedback (comments) about constructive criticism and well-delivered discussion about areas for improvement are especially valued.
[c] "In group" means the clinician is indistinguishable from the rest with respect to negative flags on confidential peer-to-peer and CRNA-to-attending evaluation questions that map to the Accreditation Council for Graduate Medical Education (ACGME) core competencies and to summative questions, such as "I am comfortable recommending this provider to care for a friend or family member."

department's compensation system and through merit-based and mission-based annual reassignment of administrative and academic time.

All members of a large organization are unique, with their own arrays of contributions to excellence along with (almost inevitably) some shortcomings. For example, **Box 2** lists yellow and red flag events, which are performance items that can largely or completely negate the value of even the most productive clinician.

The balanced scorecard recognizes this complexity and allows the departmental leadership to recognize and value all productive members of the department without a rank order list, while acknowledging different strengths and interests among the faculty.

Compensation Models for Anesthesiologists and Related Physicians

Compensation rewards desired behaviors, actions, and attributes. In turn, compensation models are heavily influenced by a worker's relation to the health care payer. At opposite ends of the spectrum, there are solo (or partnership) private practice and pure employment models. In solo and partnership private practice, an anesthesiologist's compensation is all revenue after expenses. In a full-employment model, the anesthesiologist earns a salary and the employer is fully interposed between the anesthesiologist and payers. In any model, it is almost impossible to map elements of compensation directly to each and every desired aspect of performance and capability in work. In theory, the solo private practitioner is motivated to do all the work required to optimize their practice on behalf of their patients and the organizations where they work and to use funds when necessary to self-invest in quality and process improvement. Similarly, in a full-employment model, the employing corporation might be expected to cross-subsidize performance improvement and innovation from

---

Box 2
Yellow and red flag events/characteristics (examples; not exhaustive)

Yellow flags

Recurrent late billing problems after education/counseling

Multiple focused professional practice evaluations, changing areas of concern

Multiple professionalism complaints from coworkers

Patient complaints out of proportion to group rate[a]

Disclosed substance dependence, in treatment and under management contract

Red flags[b]

Recurrent focused professional practice evaluations, same area of concern

Failure to satisfactorily complete focused professional practice evaluation

Professionalism, patient satisfaction, or preventable patient safety events that are egregious

Failure to disclose driving under the influence or other arrests

Falsification or willful failure to disclose on conflict of interest, legal actions, substance dependency, and practice-limiting condition documentation

Recurrent disruptive behavior

[a] Research from the authors' department demonstrates that after adjusting for anesthetic and patient factors, patient complaints are homogeneous across the provider group.[44]
[b] Egregious red flags may invalidate all other valuable characteristics in the balanced scorecard.

practice revenue. In actuality, there has been strong pressure in both models to reserve most or all revenue to the owners. Moreover, in a salary-only full-employment model, effort above the accepted clinical requirement can be seen as diminishing compensation per unit of effort. Thus, simple compensation models, in the setting of the current fee-for-service payment system, seem at odds with the imperative to improve the anesthesia value proposition.

Two things seem necessary to facilitate improving the value proposition: an enlightened owner/partnership willing to commit resources (ie, divert clinical revenue from clinician compensation) to service improvement and tools to motivate clinicians to do the required work (ie, components of compensation tied to work that does not generate ASA units and/or work units). To accomplish the latter, many practices now seek a middle ground, with anesthesiologists earning a base salary and participating in an organized financial incentive program designed to motivate desired behaviors as defined by leadership, group consensus, or some other mechanism. As the consolidation of anesthesiology continues, the potential for enlightened owner/partnership increases (although the jury is still out on whether this comes to pass), but more and more anesthesiologists will enter compensation arrangements with at least the potential for incentives directed to activity beyond "surfing a stool for units."

A department conveys its appreciation of individual provider value to clinicians and faculty through compensation, recognition for effective leadership, educational and scholarly effort, and a structured faculty development program. Direct compensation is an obvious vehicle. What should compensation incentive programs look like? Ordinarily, peer-reviewed literature would be used to answer a question in medical science. In 2005, 71% of respondents in a survey of academic anesthesia departments had defined incentive compensation programs, typically accounting for less than 25% of compensation.[31] However, the requirement to test a hypothesis to achieve publication has led to a strong adverse publication bias to the topic of compensation, and the literature is scant, especially for anesthesiologists. The authors conducted a review of the available literature in January, 2015, and arrived at the synopsis presented in **Table 1**. As expected for largely clinical departments, incentive compensation was biased toward clinical productivity, and these components of the plans were the best developed.

The authors' department's compensation plan follows the models in **Table 1**. Approximately two-thirds of compensation is a base salary paid for availability to schedule weekdays, holidays, call, and bedside teaching, and active participation in all departmental activities, including clinical research, quality improvement, operational improvement, and administrative work. The remaining one-third of compensation includes

- A first-dollar clinical incentive paid in proportion to the number of ASA units and relative value units (RVUs) generated and extra hours and call worked, individually calculated and awarded to each faculty member throughout the year
- An annual bonus payment tied to objective assessment of the faculty member's academic accomplishments (see **Box 1**; **Fig. 2**)
- A quarterly quality incentive bonus payment (for attainment of objective thresholds on predefined quality process measures)[40]

As a group, the departmental faculty's clinical productivity (measured as ASA units and work RVUs [wRVUs]) is consistently at or above the 90th percentile for its cohort.

The department also curates each faculty member's career in the interest of helping individual clinicians maximize their productivity and career satisfaction, while aligning with institutional goals. The process by which this is achieved is illustrated in **Fig. 2**.

Table 1
Compensation incentive programs

Year of Publication	Reference	Base Compensation (% of Total)	Performance (Clinical and Operational Performance)	Clinical Productivity	Quality (Health Care Process and Outcomes Quality)	Citizenship	Academic Productivity	Outcomes Measured – Achieved/Observed Outcome
2013	Levin LS, Gustave L. "Aligning incentives in health care: physician practice and health system partnership."[32]	80	N	wRVU	Alignment with SCIP and HCAHPS initiatives. Example was attendance of focused training program (process measure)	Billing compliance, grand rounds and faculty meeting attendance	5%; Target and outcome determined by annual negotiation with chair	Integration of hospital and departmental mission, support for research and leadership initiatives and other modern quality initiatives were rewarded. All academic, quality, and clinical productivity measures that were incentivized improved or increased. Stressed importance of alignment with institution.

(continued on next page)

Table 1
(*continued*)

Year of Publication	Reference	Base Compensation (% of Total)	Performance (Clinical and Operational Performance)	Clinical Productivity	Quality (Health Care Process and Outcomes Quality)	Citizenship	Academic Productivity	Outcomes Measured – Achieved/Observed Outcome
2013	Sakai T, Hudson M, Davis P, et al. "Integration of academic and clinical performance-based faculty compensation plans: a system and its impact on an anaesthesiology department."[33]	70	N	Measured by time units (hours); adjustments made for complexity; specifically not adjusted for wRVU	N	N	Opportunity to commit up to 80% nonclinical time for research; output measured by scoring system and was salary at risk	Clinical output and academic output increased dramatically, with clinical output increasing more. All academic faculty earned salary at risk after 1 y of implementation. Initially, composition of faculty changed: less academic faculty and more clinical faculty, this ultimately returned to baseline.
2010	Holcombe RF, Hollinger KJ. "Mission-focused, productivity-based model for sustainable support of academic hematology/oncology faculty and divisions."[34]	Yes; undisclosed	N	wRVU	N	N	Salary at risk; lectures/y; time teaching; teaching evaluations; funding, number of pubs, invited speaker	Increase in clinical productivity after first year 26%; other results not disclosed

Year	Reference							Outcome
2008	Reich DL, Galati M, Krol M, et al. "A mission-based productivity compensation model for an academic anesthesiology department."[35]	30	Points; participation in performance improvement committees; M&M coordination	ASA units (points)	Points; important institutional leadership roles	NORA points; surveys of peers; professionalism; departmental functions	Points for publication, research, education and community service assessed by departmental committee	ASA units/month increased per OR FTE (31%), as did compensation per FTE (40%). This despite stable trend in clinical productivity per anesthetizing location. Academic and educational output was preserved.
2005	Miller RD, Cohen NH. "The impact of productivity-based incentives on faculty salary-based compensation."[36]	Yes; undisclosed	N	Bonus for billable hours of availability above threshold required by base salary	N	Grand rounds attendance; Additional call availability; evening relief of residents	Residency evaluations	Clinical productivity increased mostly for junior faculty, variability in total compensation increased dramatically (within ranks), difference in compensation between ranks decreased, academic and teaching performance also increased during period of clinical incentivization, and was incentivized by nonclinical days

(continued on next page)

Table 1
(continued)

Year of Publication	Reference	Base Compensation (% of Total)	Performance (Clinical and Operational Performance)	Clinical Productivity	Quality (Health Care Process and Outcomes Quality)	Citizenship	Academic Productivity	Outcomes Measured – Achieved/Observed Outcome
2004	St Jacques PJ, Patel N, Higgins MS. "Improving anesthesiologist performance through profiling and incentives."[37]	N/A	Operational performance measured by ACT and FCOTS	N	Incentivized OR efficiency measures; compared with peers (top 20% in department received financial reward)	N	N	Performance incentives improved efficiency performance measures: ACTs, FCOTS, and decreased delays
2003	Tarquinio GT, Dittus RS, Byrne DW, et al. "Effects of performance-based compensation and faculty track on the clinical activity, research portfolio, and teaching mission of a large academic department of medicine."[38]	Yes; was set as target based on benchmark RVU; variable among faculty	N	Clinical benchmark RVUs; administrative RVUs were also assigned to other clinical leadership tasks	N	N	Bonus eligible based on funding and meeting clinical target	Billing (collections) clinical productivity, research (NIH funding and rank) increased. Faculty satisfaction with plan was directly proportional to understanding of plan and indirectly proportional to years as faculty.

| 2002 | Andreae MC, Freed GL. "Using a productivity-based physician compensation program at an academic health center: a case study."[39] | Yes; clinical target set to achieve base (70% MGMA median wRVUs) | N | wRVU generated in excess of requirement (70% MGMA median wRVUs) rewarded wRVU credit (credit reflected MGMA's $/wRVU conversion) | N | wRVU credit received for teaching efforts; residency evaluations; negotiated with chiefs and chair | N | N | 89% Of faculty had increase in clinical productivity. Clinical productivity by department increased 20% in first year, and additional 14.5% the second year. Teaching productivity was also incentivized in this study and teaching efforts were level after implementation. |

Abbreviations: ACT, anesthesia-controlled time; FCOTS, first case on-time start; FTE, full-time equivalent; HCAHPS, Hospital Consumer Assessment of Healthcare Providers and Systems; M&M, morbidity and mortality; MGMA, Medical Group Management Association; N, no; NIH, National Institutes of Health; NORA, non-OR anesthesia; SCIP, Surgical Care Improvement Project.
Data from Refs.[32–39]

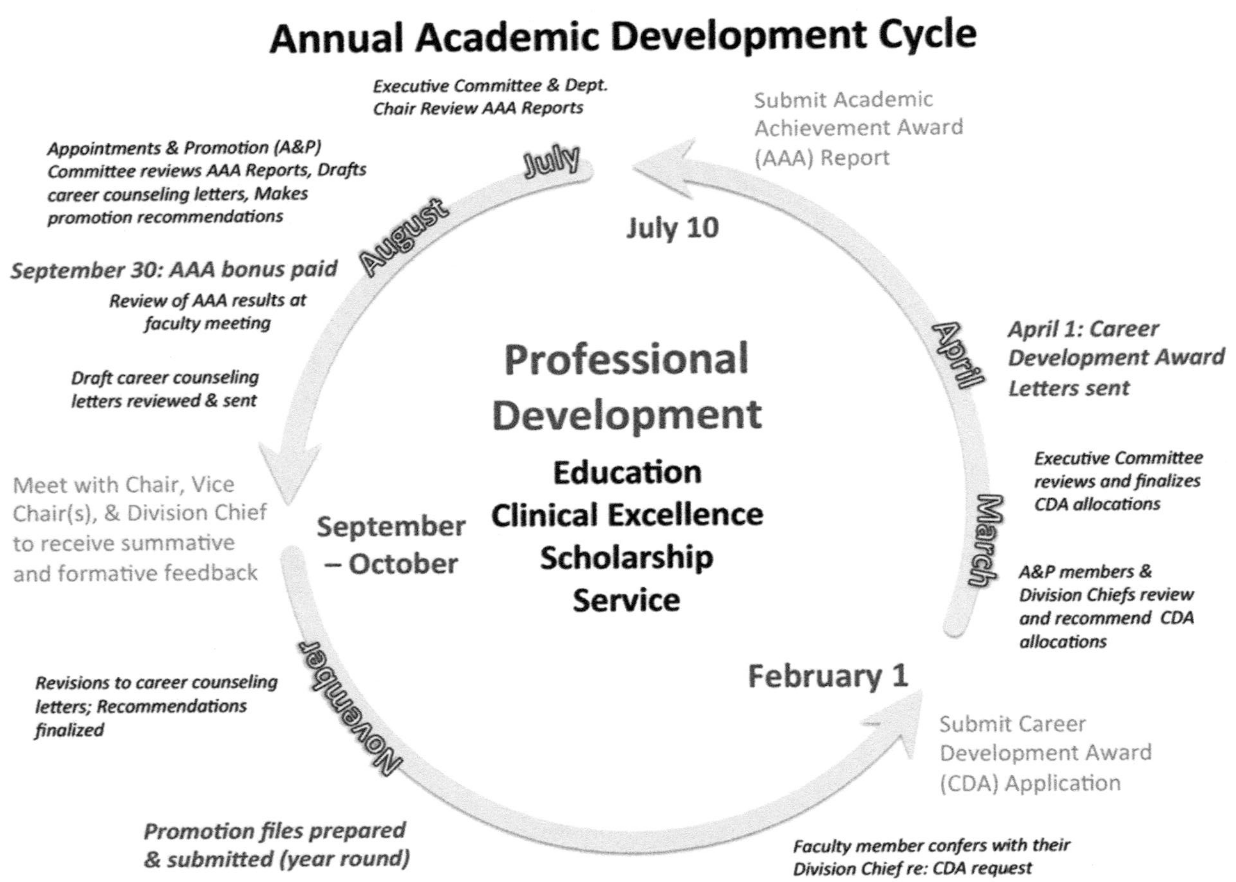

Annual Academic Development Cycle

Fig. 2. Annual faculty development and career tracking program at Vanderbilt Department of Anesthesiology. The academic year begins in July, and the key milestones are described around the outside of the circle. Major information flow between individual faculty members and departmental administration is shown in light gold; major transfers of value from the department to the faculty are shown in dark gold. The overall effect is to create an ongoing dialogue between the developing faculty and the department that keeps the faculty aligned with and developing in support of departmental missions that differentiate the departmental health care product from potential competitors.

Each year, the department conducts a mandatory application process for academic and administrative time. Each member's request for time is reviewed by departmental leadership (in this case, a committee comprising the division chiefs and vice chairs) for merit, alignment with department missions, and prior achievements (including external funding). Academic and administrative time is awarded for all departmental and institutional activities that displace clinical effort. The cost of academic and administrative time is covered primarily by cross-subsidization from clinical revenues and to a lesser extent by external funding. Academic and administrative time is adjusted upward or downward annually on the basis of this review and then constrained to fit within the department's budget. Consequently, the award of time is a demonstration of the individual clinician's nonclinical portfolio value, assessed by the established leadership of the department. Annual review of requests for academic time and individual academic accomplishments also informs the department's organized process to assess each member's readiness for academic promotion. This, in turn, drives an annual mentoring session to guide each faculty member toward promotion, and reflects increased capability of the faculty in service of the institution (and also increases compensation). Finally, the department chair retains control of approximately 1% of the total compensation pool for provision of bonuses for exemplary contributions to departmental mission in a given year.

This compensation plan gives the clinician agency over their earnings. Clinicians also have autonomy over which activities they engage in and to what extent. Operation of this system for the past 5 years has corresponded with increasing faculty accomplishment, as assessed by academic promotion (**Fig. 3**), which translates into additional faculty capabilities and leadership experience available to the institution. The departmental leadership can (and does) adjust the relative value of incentives to motivate the faculty in desired directions. Because the determinants of compensation, discretionary time, and academic promotion are all transparently displayed to the faculty, little departmental energy is expended in negotiation over any of these, which optimizes organizational efficiency.

FUTURE CONSIDERATIONS/SUMMARY

Individual-level assessment in anesthesiology is possible, using a variety of methods. Recent notable external assessments of anesthesiologists illustrate large differences in mortality and morbidity between high-performing and low-performing anesthesiologists in cardiac surgery.[41] Looking closer to home, at the clinician level to department level, a balanced scorecard approach taking in readily measurable factors is feasible, as evidenced in **Boxes 1** and **2** and **Table 1**. This assessment presupposes an anesthesiologist is part of a group, so that comparisons can be made. The strong forces driving consolidation in health care virtually assure that large group membership will become true for most anesthesiologists.

When trying to improve a product, investment is required. Most compensation plans in group practice offer at least the potential to invest some revenue in developing new capabilities to improve the group's value proposition. Large private practices and academic practices can (and do) use this strategy. Diverting revenue away from direct compensation can be viewed either as a pay reduction or as an investment in future earning opportunities. Small group and individual practices seem potentially vulnerable to the impulse to maximize clinician income by eschewing infrastructure investment. Tightly linked surgeon-anesthesiologist models do not allow resource pooling to create headroom to invest in development of individual anesthesiologists. Thus, rudimentary capability improvement activities, such as continuing medical education,

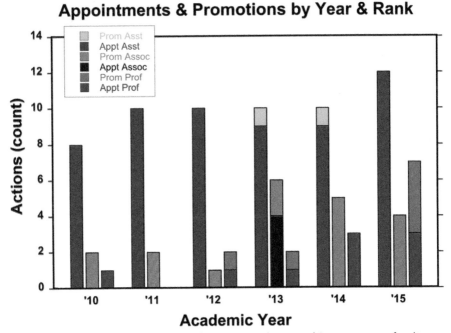

Fig. 3. The results of departmental faculty review and mentorship program on faculty promotions. Promotions and primary appointments (recruitment of new faculty) by academic rank, year on year, over 6 years' operation of the Vanderbilt Department of Anesthesiology mentorship and faculty development program. Early in the program, most appointments were at the rank of assistant professor, and promotions were to the rank of associate professor. As the program matured, assistant professor appointments continued, but promotions to senior rank (associate professor and professor) increased. Moreover, as the reputation of the department increased, recruitment into the professorial rank increased. Assoc, associate; Asst, assistant; Prof, professor; Prom, promotion; Appt, appointment.

may be viewed as competing with the opportunity to earn. Taken to extremes, solo anesthesiology practitioners may not be available to provide care to their own patients in the recovery room if they have started another case or are driving between hospitals.[42] Thus, this practice model is unlikely to survive the quality improvement expectation required to remain a viable anesthesiology product.

Compensation plans, when well designed, can motivate groups of anesthesiology clinicians to be productive on multiple axes. As consolidation continues in anesthesiology, academic and large private practice groups will become increasingly similar and share objectives for their clinicians, including clinical productivity but also engagement in institutional leadership and improvement work. Moreover, meaningful process improvement and quality improvement require the interplay of academic and business skills, such as experimental design, evaluation of results, team leadership, communication (written) of findings, leadership of implementation, and change management. To be effective, compensation plans must reward success in these areas as well as clinical productivity. Finally, compensation plans themselves must be adaptable to changing circumstances so that they can be modified to meet changing needs for recognition. In the authors' system, the development of an Anesthesia Perioperative Consult Service has reduced inpatient LOS substantially, benefiting the hospital but without generating direct ASA units or RVUs for the department. Thus, the current compensation plan will need to be modified to recognize this effort.

Individual clinician value assessment should help clinicians improve their skills across all axes of engagement, find joy and interest in their work, and maintain engagement by allowing development of mastery, autonomy, and a sense of purpose. Ideally, value assessment is an ongoing dialogue between the clinician and the department, allowing clinicians to develop their capabilities and tighten alignment with the host organization (department and host facility). Compensation is a tool to provide tangible rewards for success.

REFERENCES

1. Dexter F, Lee JD, Dow AJ, et al. A psychological basis for anesthesiologists' operating room managerial decision-making on the day of surgery. Anesth Analg 2007;105(2):430–4.
2. Kheterpal S, Tremper KK, Shanks A, et al. Workforce and finances of the United States anesthesiology training programs: 2009–2010. Anesth Analg 2011;112(6): 1480–6.
3. Sandberg WS. Barbarians at the gate. Anesth Analg 2009;109(3):695–9.
4. Available at: https://services.aamc.org/fssreports/general/generalmenu.cfm?current_survey_year=2014. Accessed April 1, 2015.
5. Kash BA, Zhang Y, Cline KM, et al. The perioperative surgical home (PSH): a comprehensive review of US and non-US studies shows predominantly positive quality and cost outcomes. Milbank Q 2014;92(4):796–821.
6. Available at: http://www.anesthesiallc.com/publications/anesthesia-industry-ealerts/229-balance-bill; http://education.asahq.org/2014/Rovenstine. Accessed April 1, 2015.
7. Levitt T. Marketing success through differentiation-of anything. Harvard Business Review. Graduate School of Business Administration, Harvard University; 1980. p. 83–91.
8. Austin TM, Lam HV, Shin NS, et al. Elective change of surgeon during the OR day has an operationally negligible impact on turnover time. J Clin Anesth 2014;26(5): 343–9.
9. Schoenmeyr T, Dunn PF, Gamarnik D, et al. A model for understanding the impacts of demand and capacity on waiting time to enter a congested recovery room. Anesthesiology 2009;110(6):1293–304.
10. Seim AR, Andersen B, Sandberg WS. Statistical process control as a tool for monitoring non-operative time. Anesthesiology 2006;105(2):370–80.
11. Seim AR, Dahl DM, Sandberg WS. Small changes in operative time can yield discrete increases in operating room throughput. J Endourol 2007;21(7):703–8.
12. Tiwari V, Furman WR, Sandberg WS. Predicting case volume from the accumulating elective operating room schedule facilitates staffing improvements. Anesthesiology 2014;121(1):171–83.
13. Cendan JC, Good M. Interdisciplinary work flow assessment and redesign decreases operating room turnover time and allows for additional caseload. Arch Surg 2006;141(1):65–9 [discussion: 70].
14. Hanss R, Buttgereit B, Tonner PH, et al. Overlapping induction of anesthesia: an analysis of benefits and costs. Anesthesiology 2005;103(2):391–400.
15. Harders M, Malangoni MA, Weight S, et al. Improving Operating Room Efficiency Through Process Redesign. Surgery 2006;140:509–16.

16. Meyer MA, Sokal SM, Sandberg W, et al. INCOMING!-a web tracking application for PACU and post-surgical patients. J Surg Res 2006;132(2):153–8.
17. Sandberg WS, Canty T, Sokal SM, et al. Financial and operational impact of a direct-from-PACU discharge pathway for laparoscopic cholecystectomy patients. Surgery 2006;140(3):372–8.
18. Sandberg WS, Daily B, Egan M, et al. Deliberate perioperative systems design improves operating room throughput. Anesthesiology 2005;103(2):406–18.
19. Seim AR, Andersen B, Berger DL, et al. The effect of direct-from-recovery room discharge of laparoscopic cholecystectomy patients on recovery room workload. Surg Innov 2006;13(4):257–64.
20. Torkki PM, Marjamaa RA, Torkki MI, et al. Use of anesthesia induction rooms can increase the number of urgent orthopedic cases completed within 7 hours. Anesthesiology 2005;103(2):401–5.
21. Stepaniak PS, Mannaerts GH, de Quelerij M, et al. The effect of the operating room coordinator's risk appreciation on operating room efficiency. Anesth Analg 2009;108(4):1249–56.
22. Ehrenfeld JM, Epstein RH, Bader S, et al. Automatic notifications mediated by anesthesia information management systems reduce the frequency of prolonged gaps in blood pressure documentation. Anesth Analg 2011;113(2):356–63.
23. Lai M, Kheterpal S. Creating a real return-on-investment for information system implementation: life after HITECH. Anesthesiol Clin 2011;29(3):413–38.
24. Lubarsky DA, Sanderson IC, Gilbert WC, et al. Using an anesthesia information management system as a cost containment tool. Description and validation. Anesthesiology 1997;86(5):1161–9.
25. O'Reilly M, Talsma A, VanRiper S, et al. An anesthesia information system designed to provide physician-specific feedback improves timely administration of prophylactic antibiotics. Anesth Analg 2006;103(4):908–12.
26. Rothman B, Sandberg WS, St Jacques P. Using information technology to improve quality in the OR. Anesthesiol Clin 2011;29(1):29–55.
27. Spring SF, Sandberg WS, Anupama S, et al. Automated documentation error detection and notification improves anesthesia billing performance. Anesthesiology 2007;106:157–63.
28. Grosse-Sundrup M, Henneman JP, Sandberg WS, et al. Intermediate acting non-depolarizing neuromuscular blocking agents and risk of postoperative respiratory complications: prospective propensity score matched cohort study. BMJ 2012;345:e6329.
29. Ehrenfeld JM, Seim AR, Berger DL, et al. Implementation of a direct-from-recovery-room discharge pathway: a process improvement effort. Surg Innov 2009;16(3):258–65.
30. Szokol JW, Stead S. The changing anesthesia economic landscape: emergence of large multispecialty practices and accountable care organizations. Curr Opin Anaesthesiol 2014;27(2):183–9.
31. Abouleish AE, Apfelbaum JL, Prough DS, et al. The prevalence and characteristics of incentive plans for clinical productivity among academic anesthesiology programs. Anesth Analg 2005;100(2):493–501.
32. Levin LS, Gustave L. Aligning incentives in health care: physician practice and health system partnership. Clin Orthop Relat Res 2013;471(6):1824–31.
33. Sakai T, Hudson M, Davis P, et al. Integration of academic and clinical performance-based faculty compensation plans: a system and its impact on an anaesthesiology department. Br J Anaesth 2013;111(4):636–50.

34. Holcombe RF, Hollinger KJ. Mission-focused, productivity-based model for sustainable support of academic hematology/oncology faculty and divisions. J Oncol Pract 2010;6(2):74–9.
35. Reich DL, Galati M, Krol M, et al. A mission-based productivity compensation model for an academic anesthesiology department. Anesth Analg 2008;107(6):1981–8.
36. Miller RD, Cohen NH. The impact of productivity-based incentives on faculty salary-based compensation. Anesth Analg 2005;101(1):195–9 [table of contents].
37. St Jacques PJ, Patel N, Higgins MS. Improving anesthesiologist performance through profiling and incentives. J Clin Anesth 2004;16(7):523–8.
38. Tarquinio GT, Dittus RS, Byrne DW, et al. Effects of performance-based compensation and faculty track on the clinical activity, research portfolio, and teaching mission of a large academic department of medicine. Acad Med 2003;78(7):690–701.
39. Andreae MC, Freed GL. Using a productivity-based physician compensation program at an academic health center: a case study. Acad Med 2002;77(9):894–9.
40. Ehrenfeld JM, Henneman JP, Peterfreund RA, et al. Ongoing professional performance evaluation (OPPE) using automatically captured electronic anesthesia data. Jt Comm J Qual Patient Saf 2012;38(2):73–80.
41. Glance LG, Kellermann AL, Hannan EL, et al. The impact of anesthesiologists on coronary artery bypass graft surgery outcomes. Anesth Analg 2015;120(3):526–33.
42. Epstein RH, Dexter F, Lopez MG, et al. Anesthesiologist staffing considerations consequent to the temporal distribution of hypoxemic episodes in the postanesthesia care unit. Anesth Analg 2014;119(6):1322–33.
43. Baker K. Determining resident clinical performance: getting beyond the noise. Anesthesiology 2011;115(4):862–78.
44. Kynes JM, Schildcrout JS, Hickson GB, et al. An analysis of risk factors for patient complaints about ambulatory anesthesiology care. Anesth Analg 2013;116(6):1325–32.

Performance Measurement to Demonstrate Value

Joseph A. Hyder, MD, PhD[a],*, James R. Hebl, MD[b]

KEYWORDS

- Performance measurement • Quality metrics • Perioperative value
- Reliability adjustment • Risk adjustment • National quality forum

KEY POINTS

- Performance measures are used within and across institutions to compare the quality and efficiency of care and determine payment. Different measures matter to different stakeholders.
- Performance measures include structure, process, outcome, and efficiency measure types, each with characteristic advantages and disadvantages as tools for value demonstration.
- The Centers for Medicare and Medicaid Services and the National Quality Forum have libraries of performance measures used to compare and encourage high-value care, but these measures have important limitations.
- In addition to externally reported measures, internally designed and reported performance measures can be used to demonstrate and encourage high-value care.

MATCHING MESSAGE TO MEASURES: WHO IS DEMONSTRATING VALUE TO WHOM?

Perioperative care has numerous stakeholders—surgeons, nurses, hospitals, private and public payers, our own anesthesia colleagues, and, of course, patients. Which performance measures are invoked as the best evidence of high-value care will vary according to who is asking whom for the evidence (**Table 1**). Definitions of perioperative value and emphasis on different measures will be specific to the organizational structure of a care delivery system (integrated or not), the nature of payment (such as bundled or fee for service), and the extent to which patients are centered in the perioperative process. Articles in this issue emphasize, implicitly or explicitly, different performance measures as evidence of high-value care. As anesthesiologists, we are responsible to all stakeholders to demonstrate the value of the care we provide.

Disclosures: The authors have no disclosures.
[a] Division of Critical Care Medicine, Department of Anesthesiology, Kern Center for the Science of Health Care Delivery, Mayo Clinic, 200 1st Street Southwest, Rochester, MN 55905, USA;
[b] Department of Anesthesiology, Mayo Clinic, 200 1st Street Southwest, Rochester, MN 55905, USA
* Corresponding author.
E-mail address: joseph.a.hyder@gmail.com

Anesthesiology Clin 33 (2015) 679–696
http://dx.doi.org/10.1016/j.anclin.2015.07.007
1932-2275/15/$ – see front matter © 2015 Elsevier Inc. All rights reserved.
anesthesiology.theclinics.com

Table 1
Who is demonstrating value to whom? The anesthesiologist's turn to demonstrate value

Anesthesiologists Demonstrating Value to Whom	General Example

Surgeons	Operating room efficiency
	    Case cancellations
	    On-time starts
	    Rapid turnover
	Patient satisfaction and medical outcomes

Hospitals	Timely service across all service lines Service for undercompensated service lines Ability to compete for payer incentives
Payers	Resource utilization Predetermined measures
Patients	Patient satisfaction and medical outcome Costs of care

One aim of health care innovation is to improve the clarity and alignment of care goals so that all stakeholders share the same concept of value and can strive to achieve complementary, if not identical, empirical definitions of value.

In this article, we describe the basics of performance measures as they are used to demonstrate perioperative value care. We address the approach used by the Centers for Medicare and Medicaid Services (CMS) in which performance measures are externally reported and linked to payment in an effort to drive value. We then present an example of internally reported performance measurement from a large, multispecialty group practice. For all examples, performance measurement as strategy for demonstrating value will require a tailored approach for changes in measures, employment models, and payment systems.

HOW IS VALUE MEASURED IN HEALTH CARE? INTRODUCTION TO STRUCTURE, PROCESS, OUTCOME AND EFFICIENCY MEASURES

Performance measures in health care are commonly placed into 1 of 3 categories—structure, process, and outcome. These categories were described in 1966 in the Donabedian Model used to assess the quality of medical care.[1] Over time, the quality movement, which invented these categories, evolved into the patient safety movement and, more recently, into a business case for quality improvement (ie, value improvement)[2] with a customer-commodity orientation called *patient-centered care*. The nature of the structure-process-outcome categories has similarly evolved to include a new category commonly referred to as *efficiency*.[3] Some of the demarcations among measure types have blurred, as we will see, but the categories remain important. These measure types have important advantages and shortcoming as tools to demonstrate and improve value.

STRUCTURAL MEASURES: LARGELY A RELIC OF THE PAST

Structural performance measures may include participation in a data registry, 24-hour in-house coverage or board certification by physicians. Although they often have the advantages of ease of measurement and the ring of significance, structural measures may be the least useful markers of quality or value. These measures have become less common among measures used by the CMS or the National Quality Forum (NQF).

PROCESS MEASURES
Simple, Actionable Targets for Improvement

Process measures focus on what is done to the patient, such as timely administration of antibiotics or postoperative removal of a urinary catheter. These measures are intended to capture best practices and improve quality through the standardization of care. Process measures are simple and inexpensive to track. At a local level, they can serve as clear targets for improvement. Comparing performance, whether over time, between operating rooms, or across hospitals, may be done meaningfully with exclusions rather than risk adjustment. Because of their alignment with best practices, demonstrating success with process measures can give the impression of achieving high-value care.

Tenuous Links to Value

Despite these advantages, process measures have critical shortcomings. Numerous examples of best practices have later been demonstrated to be inconsequential or even harmful to patients. This is particularly troubling because targeting processes rather than results has the potential to disrupt the alignment of goals for hospitals, physicians, and patients. From the organizational–cultural perspective, this disruption cannot be underestimated. Another important criticism of process measures is that they focus on "what the doctor does" rather than "how the patient does," and this emphasis is not patient centered or quality focused.

Process measures, strictly speaking, do not measure the variables that make up value: quality, patient experience, and costs. In some instances, process measures have excellent face value as proxies for costs or quality. For example, operating room turnover time may seem to be an excellent process measure given its face value and simplicity of tracking compared with actual operating room costs. However, as a later example demonstrates, turnover time may be a poor indicator of efficiency in a surgical suite.

Although process measures may be poor targets for demonstrating the value of care, their simplicity and utility as specific, actionable targets will make them an irreplaceable part of value improvement efforts for years to come. These measures are likely to remain relevant as value surrogates as well, particularly for smaller practices lacking the resources and expertise necessary to implement a system to track and compare outcomes or efficiencies.

Process Measures to Demonstrate Value: Geisinger Health System "ProvenCare"

An example of the use of process measures as value targets is the Geisinger Health System "ProvenCare" strategy for cardiac surgery. Beginning in 2005, Geisinger derived 40 process measures from 20 guidelines in the American College of Cardiology/American Heart Association 2004 Guideline Update for Coronary Artery Bypass Graft (CABG) Surgery.[4] At the same time, Geisinger offered payers a single-payment for CABG surgery to include all costs of care from preoperative evaluation to 90-days of postoperative care. Surgeons' pay was linked to performance on the 40-item checklist but not to outcomes. Over 3 months, compliance with the 40-item checklist increased from 59% to 100% with evidence of long-term adherence rate of 100%. This extreme success with 40 process measures translated to minimal measured changes in value. Clinical outcomes did not differ other than a small increase in home discharge. Hospital charges decreased by a reported 5%.[5,6] No reports have disclosed the costs of the design, implementation, or tracking of this intensive process-oriented system.

Process Measures to Demonstrate Value: Surgical Checklists

An emerging process of care from surgical literature that is making itself into a process measure is the surgical safety checklist. Such a checklist was found to decrease mortality in a trial,[7] but in a subsequent observational study, implementation of the checklist was found to have no effect on surgical mortality.[8] The effect that a process measure may have on outcomes may be better estimated from the observation study.[9,10] The discrepancy between compliance with processes of care and value is critical to appreciate and re-evaluate if process measures are to be used to measure value. Regardless, care checklists for perioperative handoffs, or transitions of care, are being considered by CMS,[11] but these specific checklists do not have evidence for a link with either outcomes or costs.

OUTCOME MEASURES
Traditional Means to Demonstrate Value

Patient outcomes, along with costs, are the key components of value. Outcome measures directly address "how the patient does" and are increasingly common among the performance measures used by CMS and the NQF to benchmark care. Outcomes such as complications or death are undesirable for all stakeholders, have excellent face value for all stakeholders in perioperative care, and are costly.[12,13] For these reasons, outcome measures focused on morbidity and mortality are commonly used by CMS, the NQF, and other high-profile quality comparison organizations.[3] For the sake of demonstrating high-value care, however, outcome measures using complications and death may make for poor performance measures.

Outcome Measures Have Important Limitations

The major shortcoming of outcome measures are (1) morbidity and mortality outcome measures have a limited ability to capture what matter most to patients, (2) traditional outcome endpoints have significant methodologic limitations when used for benchmarking (see later discussion), and (3) outcome measures do not inform providers how to go about improving value. When measuring the value of care, the most important outcome to measure is the outcome that matters to patients.[14] Nearly all outcome measures used by the CMS or NQF focus on postoperative harms, specifically complications or mortality.[15,16] By contrast, patients' motivations for surgery are nearly always focused on postoperative benefits such as increased functionality, decreased pain, and prolonged lives well beyond the 30-day or 90-day windows used in current outcome measures.

Evolution and Innovation of Outcome Measures: Scoring What Went Right

For outcome measures to be meaningful as value targets, they will need to maintain face validity to stakeholders while becoming more diverse. This process is well underway. Current outcome measures in the NQF for cataract surgery track return of good vision, and measures for obstetric care track delivery of a healthy newborn.[15] These are clearly outcomes that matter to patients and markers of high-value care. Another example of this innovation in outcome measures is for hip replacement. Although CMS already has 2 existing measures that track readmissions and complications, CMS is proposing a new outcome measure for hip replacement that would track patients' functional statuses 90 days before surgery and 180 to 270 days postoperatively. This new kind of outcome measure, which may focus on what patients do want from surgery rather than what patients don't want, has great potential for demonstrating the value of care provided.

Evolution and Innovation of Outcome Measures: Scoring Patient Experience

Another example of innovation in outcome measurement is the increase of patient experience as an outcome. Patients and payers have emphasized that patients' attitudes about their care are important value targets. Multiple current and proposed perioperative outcome measures address the patient experience. More than simply "pain scores," these measures are psychometrically validated questionnaires that intend to capture diverse aspects of the patient experience. In addition to the Hospital Consumer Assessment of Healthcare Providers and Systems (CAHPS), new tools, more specific to surgical care, have been developed and gained attention in the last 5 years. A Surgical Care Survey-CAHPS tool is available and addresses satisfaction with surgeons, nurses, and anesthesiologists (https://www.facs.org/advocacy/quality/cahps).[17] One current NQF performance measure would require Surgical-CAHPS for reporting. Notably, the subset of items used in this measure does not address any aspects of anesthesia care.[3,18] In addition, the Ambulatory Surgical Center Quality Collaboration developed a questionnaire specifically for ambulatory surgical patients that addresses the patient experience, communication, and comfort, high-value aspects of both anesthesia and surgical care.[19] It should be noted that outcome measures for patient experience, like other outcome measures, may be risk adjusted, as detailed below.[20,21]

Complications and Quality May Not Correlate

Among outcome measures, those focusing on morbidity and mortality have the longest track record and are the most commonly represented outcome measures used for benchmarking. Despite their widespread use as quality markers, some important practical and methodologic limitations undermine their use as definitive measures of quality. One key limitation is that complications are prone to measurement error. Although clinical registry data may track complications more accurately than administrative data,[22] neither administrative nor clinical registry data meaningfully track the severity of most complications or the incidence of complication cascades, which are likely to be critical determinants of perioperative value.[23] In addition, many outcome measures are designed around a suite of complications, and quality is tracked by the occurrence of any one or more complications from the suite. Each complication in the suite, such as urinary tract infection or reoperation, is likely to have different implications for quality and value. Coupled with lack of data on complication severity, this measurement error challenges the utility of many outcome measures as measures of quality or value.

The Case of Venous Thromboembolism as a Quality Measure

Many outcome measures have included venous thromboembolism as a marker for postoperative quality.[15] Only recently has important work found that the incidence of postoperative venous thromboembolism does not seem to reflect hospital quality.[24] Rather, it reflects patient risk and provider suspicion for and approach to the diagnosis of the condition. Those hospitals and physicians with the greatest vigilance for venous thromboembolism would be penalized for their acumen.[25] This example illustrates an important gap between outcome measures and value measures.

Statistical Challenges to Meaningful Outcome Comparisons

When benchmarking or comparing providers in terms of quality, outcome measures require risk adjustment to ensure accurate comparison. Hospitals caring for sicker patients may reasonably be expected to have worse outcomes and more costly care than hospitals caring for healthier patients. The statistical methods used to adjust for differences in patient mix have matured considerably over the decades; however, there remains no gold standard for risk adjustment, and methods to adjust for case mix are in the early stages of development.[26–28]

In addition to the problem of risk adjustment, outcome measures face another statistical limitation, commonly called *reliability*. Reliability can be thought of as the signal-to-noise ratio in which measurement variability caused by true performance difference is the signal and variability caused by measurement error is the noise. Uncommon outcomes, such as mortality after noncardiac surgery, and uncommon surgeries, such as some thoracic surgeries, are too rare to permit meaningful comparisons across hospitals. Recent work has found that even common complications after common surgeries may suffer from inadequate statistical reliability.[29] For example, case volumes for colorectal surgery are adequate at only a quarter of US hospitals to permit the use of surgical site infection as a statistically reliable outcome measure.[30] Thus, even an outcome measure as seemingly common as surgical site infection after colorectal surgery may be a poor target for demonstrating value.

Longer-term Outcomes for Anesthesiologist to Demonstrate Value

High-value care may depend on achieving a surgical goal and limiting interaction with the medical system, such as prolonged lengths of stay and hospital readmissions. Although anesthesiologists may debate the contribution of anesthesia care to these endpoints, a common reason for readmission is wound infection, which starts in the operating room and may be reduced by intraoperative anesthesia therapies, including antibiotic administration and normothermia.[31,32] Moreover, as anesthesiologists take higher-profile roles in perioperative management, these longer-term outcomes may have greater face validity. Integration of care across the arc of a surgical episode and the ownership of longer-term outcomes would provide great potential for anesthesiologists to demonstrate value through performance measurement.

Challenges with Longer-term Outcomes to Demonstrate Value

Hospital length of stay and hospital readmissions may be attractive outcome measures for demonstrating value. These measures address issues of complication severity and heterogeneity and would have good face value for patients and hospitals. Currently, only a few NQF outcome measures have used length of stay or readmission.[15] A measure built around length of stay would be suboptimal when hospital disposition is strongly influenced by social rather more than medical issues, if such measure encourages premature hospital discharge or if payment schemes require a minimum length of stay for full payment.[6] Alternatives such as hospital-free days have not been evaluated. Readmissions may have poor measurement properties for comparing hospitals.[33,34] Moreover, surgical readmissions are frequently made at hospitals other than the hospital where the operation occurred.[35,36] Thus, such a measure may be challenging to track outside of CMS or highly integrated, even closed, care settings.

Can Single Hospitals Benefit from Using Outcome Measures to Demonstrate Value?

When outcome measures are used to demonstrate value, their management requires significant resources and expertise. Rather than undertake this internally, many hospitals rely on CMS or clinical data registries to track and report outcomes for them. The real costs of participation in clinical data registries, however, may run into hundreds of thousands of dollars per year, not including additional fees to participate in anesthesia-related components, as are offered by the Society for Thoracic Surgeons

National Database.[37] Although groups such as the American College of Surgeons have made a business case for participation in data registries, recent evidence shows that hospitals participating in such efforts do not achieve quality improvements that are different from hospitals that do not participate.[38,39] The impetus for participation in outcome measurement may not be a simple business case for value but avoidance of financial consequences of nonparticipation imposed by public and private payers.

To demonstrate changes in outcomes as part of a value argument, some hospitals have used data describing year-to-year outcomes, benchmarked by CMS or clinical data registries. This approach has been used successfully for specific quality interventions.[40,41] It should be done with caution, however. Not only can different benchmarking programs provide seemingly contradictory estimations for outcome measures,[42] but the statistical methods used to track outcomes can generate inaccurate results when applied to single hospitals.

Current benchmarking methods use shrinkage or reliability adjustment wherein performance at individual hospitals is intentionally biased toward or away from the average performance for all hospitals.[43-45] This approach is intended to permit the inclusion of small-volume hospitals and improve rankability, and it does both.[46] However, this method may result in a hospital's relative performance changing from year to year only because of changes in surgical volume and not changes in event rates. If an institution is using the observed-to-expected ratio to track outcomes performance, then conclusions about quality change may be incorrect because of shrinkage adjustment rather than true performance changes. Single-center or small-volume hospitals using these data as their primary means to demonstrate quality will be subject to the whims of measurement error and methods.

Additional Considerations About Outcome Measures and Value

Although outcome measures may be important for demonstrating value, only rarely will they provide identifiable strategies for improving value. More innovative outcome measures will push value measurement to include longer postoperative windows as with hospital-free days, readmissions, and extended windows to assess postoperative functional outcomes. Anesthesiologists may interpret these changes as threatening and as a de-emphasis on the value of anesthesia care. There is evidence to the contrary. The perioperative outcomes that lead to readmission are diverse but commonly include wound infection and ileus.[47] Anesthesiologists, in the operating room and as part of perioperative management, oversee therapies such as antibiotics, intravenous fluids, normothermia, and multimodal analgesia that may affect the rates of these complications and others.[48] Moreover, readmissions seem to be more common when postoperative care is more fragmented.[35] The movement by anesthesiologists to integrate care in the Perioperative Surgical Home may be a valuable strategy to improve outcomes, including long-term measures of what went right. Outcome measures will be critical to demonstrating the value of perioperative care.

EFFICIENCY MEASURES
More than an Old Idea with a New Name

As part of the evolution from quality to value, the concept of efficiency measure has been brought to the foreground. This measure type aims to address the costs of care more directly than structure, process, or outcome measures. Efficiency measures may be designed to have features of either process measures or outcome measures and would assume many of the corresponding advantages and disadvantages described previously. For example, one CMS efficiency measure that is more like a process measure tracks the use of cardiac imaging before low-risk noncardiac surgery. Another CMS efficiency measure that is more akin to an outcome measure compares risk-adjusted costs for specific surgeries across the perioperative episode.[3]

Great Promise for Local Solutions to Demonstrate Value

For anesthesiologists, surgeons, and hospitals, some efficiency measures have long been used internally to track resource use and costs. These measures, particularly when crafted without a need for risk adjustment, hold great potential as an approach to demonstrate value in perioperative care. They may be crafted to meet local needs, such as excessive preoperative laboratory testing, internal medicine consultations, use of high-cost medications with generic equivalents, or whatever perceived inefficiency may benefit from targeting in a specific setting. When these measures are designed as process measures, they often entail only a small measurement burden and do not necessarily require risk adjustment, although appropriate case selection is important. It is important that efficiency measures are not oversimplified or conflated with operating room efficiency, such as turnover times. These matters deserve more detailed assessment to demonstrate value, as we present below.

Costs of Care and Reporting of Efficiency

Some efficiency measures specifically address the costs of an episode of care. Even when costs of care or risk-adjusted costs of care are used to demonstrate value, it is important to explicitly define what costs mean. Just as demonstrating value depends on to whom the demonstration is made, costs vary by subject. Costs may be defined as payment made by CMS, payment received from CMS, the true costs for a hospital to deliver care, indirect costs including lost productivity, or the costs incurred by patients for their care inclusive of suffering, lost work, and so forth. The context of care and stakeholder demanding value will determine which definition of cost is most relevant. At the national level, CMS has specified risk-adjusted costs as a publicly reportable performance measure. For anesthesiologists aiming to demonstrate value, the implications and opportunities to demonstrate value with publicly reported costs data have not been investigated. Not only is the measurement science for costs of care relatively immature, but the reported CMS costs do not reflect the institutional costs of care. All stakeholders will be well served to place patients' costs first when considering the costs of care.

Managing Performance Measures to Achieve High-value Care

Although measure type (structure, process, outcome, efficiency) is important, measure governance can be even more important when using measures to benchmark or improve value. The NQF and CMS, the 2 dominant organizations using performance measures nationally, have adopted practices for management of portfolios of performance measures that improve their utility. These management practices are applicable in local settings as well. One practice is to permit a period before potential adoption of a measure for open commentary on the measure from diverse stakeholders. Stakeholders would, of course, include nurses, surgeons, anesthesiologists, operating room staff, pharmacists, and patients. Another valuable practice is to approve measures for preset trial periods or for time-limited approval. This strategy has multiple advantages. Scheduled re-evaluation permits straightforward rejection of measures that may no longer represent best practices or have a newly discovered measurement compromise. In addition, if significant performance improvements make a measure obsolete, it may be retired or replaced.[49]

Another strategy to maximize the utility of performance measures and balance quality and costs is to construct measures in pairs or composites of multiple measures. This practice can use performance measures to target performance aims across all components of value: outcomes, patient experience, and costs. Such a strategy can potentially avoid unintended consequences of a myopic measure. The use of composite measures has been the practice adopted by CMS for many payment-based performance measures discussed below.

PUBLIC REPORTING TO DRIVE HIGH-VALUE CARE AND DETERMINE PAYMENT
Pay for Performance Measurement in Centers for Medicare and Medicaid Services

Half of all health care costs in the United States is paid by government entities.[50] The federal government, specifically CMS, has advanced the scope of public reporting and tightened the link between performance measures and payment. It is estimated that nearly 10% of all Medicare payments will be linked to performance measures by the year 2017.[3] CMS has established numerous and diverse mechanisms that link performance measures and payment specifically for perioperative care or care that may include perioperative care. The scope of these programs is vast, and programs may interact, or overlap, with each other. Payment programs linked to performance measurement target physicians as individuals, small groups, and large groups. Others target hospitals providing inpatient care, systems providing outpatient care, and Accountable Care Organizations. The interaction among payment programs is not currently designed to be consistent. For instance, quality reporting requirements and associated payment modifications differ for ambulatory surgical centers (ASCs) and hospital outpatient surgical departments.[51]

Overview of Centers for Medicare and Medicaid Services Value-based Payment Programs

Here we summarize some features of CMS performance-based payment programs that use performance measures of relevance to perioperative care. Critical features of these programs will change over time, and definitive details may be found through the CMS Web site. Features that are known to change include the specific performance measures making up these programs, the relative weighting of performance measure in determining ranking, and the financial consequences of nonreporting and performance. Some programs rank, report, and reward based on performance alone, whereas others include improvement as part of ranking and payment. Elements of these programs are controversial because of problematic performance measures, double jeopardy of overlapping measures in multiple programs, and disproportionate penalties for specific hospital types, such as large teaching hospitals[52,53] (**Fig. 1, Table 2**).

Physician Quality Reporting System

Certain features unify the performance-based payment programs and should be addressed by anesthesiologists aiming to demonstrate the value of anesthesia care. For some anesthesiologists, the most important links between performance and payment will be those that are at the level of physicians and groups, such as the Physician Quality Reporting System (PQRS). To participate in PQRS, an anesthesiologist must participate in a Qualified Clinical Data Registry (QCDR) such as the National Anesthesia Clinical Outcomes Registry. The reporting rules for eligible professionals are complex and designed to change from year to year, as are the financial implications of compliance. For instance, eligible professionals must report 9 or more measures that address 3 or more National Quality Strategy domains, which include patient

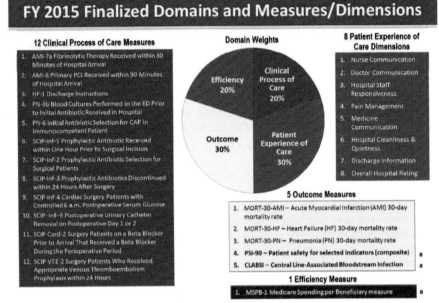

Fig. 1. Overview of CMS Hospital Value-based Purchasing Program, 2015. [a]New measure for the Fiscal Year 2015 program that was not in the Fiscal Year 2014 program. (*From* Medicare Learning Network. National provider call: hospital value-based purchasing. Centers for Medicare & Medicaid Services, March 4, 2013. Available at: http://www.cms.gov/outreach-and-education/outreach/npc/downloads/hospvbp_fy15_npc_final_03052013_508.pdf. Accessed July 14, 2015.)

safety, patient and caregiver experience, care coordination, clinical care, population health, and efficiency and cost reduction. Two or more measures must be outcomes measures. Physicians must report each measure for 50% or more of patients, regardless of the patients' Medicare status. Eligible professionals in groups fewer than 10 would be exempt from penalties. An illustration of measures for anesthesia care process, outcome, and patient experience measure types is found in **Table 3**.[54] The complexity of reporting may be matched by the financial consequences of noncompliance. Anesthesiologists may benefit from or even require third-party expertise to achieve compliance with PQRS.

Demonstrating Value Beyond Same-specialty Measures

Participation in PQRS may permit anesthesiologists to maintain payment and compare performance with other anesthesiologists. For some anesthesiologists, this may be adequate as a demonstration of their value, whether to patients, hospitals, or surgeons. More likely, the performance measures currently available will be inadequate for these purposes.[16] For the reasons discussed above, the processes and outcomes currently available are unlikely to differentiate average and high-value care to diverse stakeholders. Anesthesiologists may wish to engage with hospitals and surgeons to consider improving performance on the publicly reported measures that these stakeholders report to CMS. This approach would provide a stronger base for demonstrating value and fulfill one aim of CMS payment programs, which is to incentivize high-value care through better alignment of provider incentives and coordination of care.[55]

Table 2
Overview of CMS performance and payment programs

	Year		
	2015	2016	2017
Hospital-acquired Conditions Reduction Program			
Domain 1			
Composite of PSIs[a]	x	x	x
Domain 2			
Central line–associated blood stream infection	x	x	x
Catheter-associated urinary tract infection	x	x	x
Surgical site infection (colorectal and hysterectomy)	—	x	x
Methicillin-resistant *Staphylococcus aureus* infection rate	—	—	x
Clostridium difficile infection rate	—	—	x
Hospital Readmission Reduction Program			
Primary diagnosis			
Acute myocardial infarction	x	x	x
Heart failure	x	x	x
Pneumonia	x	x	x
Total hip or knee arthroplasty	x	x	x
Chronic obstructive pulmonary disease	x	x	x
Coronary artery bypass graft	—	—	x
ASC Quality Reporting			
Patient burn (ASC-1)	x	x	x
Patient fall (ASC-2)	x	x	x
Wrong surgery[b] (ASC-3)	x	x	x
Hospital transfer/admission (ASC-4)	x	x	x
Prophylactic intravenous antibiotic timing (ASC-5)	x	x	x
Safe surgery checklist use (ASC-6)	—	x	x
Facility volume data on selected ASC procedures	—	x	x
Influenza vaccination coverage among health care staff	—	—	x

Abbreviation: PSI, patient safety indicator.

[a] For 2015, the PSIs include PSI-3 (pressure ulcer rate), PSI-6 (iatrogenic pneumothorax), PSI-7 (central venous catheter blood stream infection rate), PSI-8 (postoperative hip fracture rate), PSI-12 (postoperative venous thromboembolism rate), PSI-13 (postoperative sepsis rate), PSI-14 (wound dehiscence rate), and PSI-15 (accidental puncture or laceration during a procedure).
[b] Wrong site, side, patient, procedure, implant.
Data from Department of Health and Human Services, Centers for Medicare & Medicaid Services. FY 2015 IPPS Final Rule. 79 Federal Register 102 (August 22, 2014) 49853–50536; and Association of American Medical Colleges. Hospital acquired condition (HAC) reduction program, September 29, 2014. Available at: https://www.aamc.org/download/405936/data/aamcfy2015hacreduction programtothepoint.pdf. Accessed July 14, 2015.

Alternative Centers for Medicare and Medicaid Services Programs for Demonstrating Value

Under the Affordable Care Act, the government pays for medical care according to value-based payment (VBP) incentives. These VBP programs are diverse and include Hospital VBP, Ambulatory Surgical Center VBP, the Hospital Readmission Reduction Program, and the Hospital Acquired Conditions Reduction Program. These programs

Table 3
Types of performance measure in perioperative care

Measure Type	Explanation/Example	Approach to Comparisons	Major Weaknesses	Major Strengths
Structure	Static description of components of care Board certification by providers	None	Limited association with value	Simple to measure
Process	What is done to the patient Percentage of patients receiving antibiotics within 60 minutes of incision	Exclusion/ Inclusion criteria	Limited association with outcomes or value Potential to encourage inappropriate care	Easy to measure Provide clear targets for process improvement
Outcome	How the patient does Postoperative wound infection within 30-days	Risk- and reliability-adjustment	Outcomes are not always quality Statistical adjustments make meaningful comparisons difficult	Strong face validity with stakeholders Come closer to measuring quality
Efficiency	Resource utilization Cardiac imaging prior to low-risk noncardiac surgery	Variable	Difficulty measure Similar to process and outcome measures	Focus specifically on resource utilization and costs that make up value

contain elements that involve perioperative care, whether directly or indirectly, and are summarized in **Table 4**.

In the Hospital Outpatient Quality Reporting Program, hospitals submit data for approximately 27 quality measures in 2015, although additional reporting requirements have not been set for future years (**Table 5**). The measures under the Hospital Outpatient Quality Reporting Program are diverse but, as with the other CMS programs, include anesthesia-related measures. These measures include the use of a Safe Surgery Checklist, Hospital Outpatient Volume Data on Selected Outpatient Surgical Procedures, and Cardiac Imaging for Preoperative Risk Assessment for Non-Cardiac Low-Risk Surgery. What stands out among the diversity of performance measures used by CMS in this program and others is that, among all medical and surgical specialties, anesthesiology may have the greatest potential impact of these measures globally. The anesthesiologist may meaningfully affect preoperative, intraoperative, and postoperative care of all surgical patients from all surgical specialties as well as critically ill patients requiring imaging and those requiring sedation for procedures performed by radiologists, cardiologists, pulmonologists, and gastroenterologists.

The extent to which CMS payment modification is part of a value demonstration will be determined, in part, by the nature of the financial relationships linking anesthesiologists, hospitals, and surgeons. Regardless, performance on specific measures is linked to payment, and performance measures may be used demonstrate value in these simple terms.

A CASE STUDY OF PERFORMANCE MEASURE TO DRIVE VALUE AT MAYO CLINIC

Performance measures are valuable for demonstrating value internally and externally. For internal demonstrations, process measures and intermediate outcomes (such as

Table 4
Performance measures for anesthesiologists eligible for the PQRS within the National Anesthesia Clinical Outcomes Registry

Type	Title	Source
Process	Preoperative β-blocker in patients with isolated CABG surgery	PQRS
Process	Prevention of central venous catheter-related bloodstream infections	PQRS
Process	Documentation of current medications	PQRS
Process	Perioperative temperature management	PQRS
Process	Smoking screening and cessation intervention	PQRS
Process	Surgical risk assessment and communication	PQRS
Patient experience	Pain brought under control within 48 h	PQRS
Process	Postoperative transfer of care protocol from OR to PACU	QCDR
Process	Post-op transfer of care protocol from OR to ICU	QCDR
Process	Prevention of postoperative nausea and vomiting, adults	QCDR
Process	Prevention of postoperative vomiting, pediatrics	QCDR
Outcome	Composite procedural safety for central line placement	QCDR
Outcome	Successful completion of planned procedure (composite safety)	QCDR
Outcome	OR/PACU cardiac arrest rate	QCDR
Outcome	OR/PACU all-cause mortality	QCDR
Outcome	PACU reintubation rate	QCDR
Patient experience	PACE acute pain management success	QCDR
Patient experience	Composite anesthesia patient satisfaction	QCDR

Abbreviations: OR, operating room; PACU, postanesthesia care unit.

unplanned admission to the intensive care unit) may be most realistic. More commonly, efficiency measures are targeted for value demonstration. For internal reporting, these measures may be tailored for local priorities and more carefully linked to specific cost centers such as number of full-time equivalent personnel, overtime hours by operating room staff, case volumes, and revenue per case. Here we present an example of performance measurement to drive and demonstrate value at a single, large-volume, tertiary referral hospital.[56]

Collaboration, Cooperation, and Coordination

At Mayo Clinic in Rochester, Minnesota in 2008, an institutional initiative was undertaken to improve efficiency of surgical care through a global assessment of patient flow from the surgical consult through postoperative recovery. This labor-intensive endeavor required active participation from diverse stakeholders including surgeons from a dozen specialties and subspecialties, anesthesiologists, hospitalists, certified registered nurse anesthetists, logisticians, financial specialists, and registered nurses across the surgical spectrum. Using Lean and Six Sigma methodologies (approaches discussed in this issue) and value-stream mapping, the effort identified 5 theoretic areas for improvement as follows: reduction in unplanned surgical volume variation, streamlining the preoperative process, reducing nonoperative time (ie, turnover time), reduction in collection of redundant patient information, and employee engagement. Each work stream was assigned to task forces to undergo analysis and coordination with other work streams to improve care processes. After coordination, performance measures were created to assess the value of changes in surgical processes.

Table 5
Hospital outpatient quality reporting quality measures

OP-1	Median time to fibrinolysis
OP-2	Fibrinolytic therapy received within 30 min of ED arrival
OP-3	Median time to transfer to another facility for acute coronary intervention
OP-4	Aspirin at arrival
OP-5	Median time to electrocardiogram
OP-6	Timing of antibiotic prophylaxsis
OP-7	Prophylactic antibiotic selection for surgical patients
OP-8	MRI lumbar spine for low back pain
OP-9	Mammography follow-up rates
OP-10	Abdomen CT use of contrast material
OP-11	Thorax CT use of contrast material
OP-12	The ability for providers with HIT to receive laboratory data electronically directly into their ONC-certified EHR system as discrete searchable data
OP-13	Cardiac imaging for preoperative risk assessment for non-cardiac low-risk surgery
OP-14	Simultaneous use of brain CT and sinus CT
OP-15	Use of brain CT in the ED for atraumatic headache—REPORTING POSTPONED[a]
OP-17	Tracking clinical results between visits
OP-18	Median time from ED arrival to ED departure for discharged ED patients
OP-19	Transition record with specified elements received by discharged patients—MEASURE REMOVED[b]
OP-20	Door to diagnostic evaluation by a qualified medical professional
OP-21	ED—Median time to pain management for long bone fracture
OP-22	ED—Patient left without being seen
OP-23	ED—Head CT or MRI scan results for acute ischemic stroke or hemorrhagic stroke who received head CT or MRI scan interpretation within 45 min of arrival
OP-25	Safe surgery checklist use
OP-26	Hospital outpatient volume data on selected outpatient surgical procedures
OP-27	Influenza vaccination coverage among health care personnel (reported on the National Healthcare Safety Network Web site)
OP-29	Endoscopy/polyp surveillance: appropriate follow-up interval for normal colonoscopy in average-risk patients
OP-30	Endoscopy/polyp surveillance: colonoscopy interval for patients with a history of adenomatous polyps—Avoidance of inappropriate use
OP-31	Cataracts—Improvement in patient's visual function within 90 d after cataract surgery

Abbreviations: CT, computed tomography; EHR, electronic health record; HIT, health information technology; ONC, Office of the National Coordinator for Health Information Technology.

[a] Public reporting of measure OP-15 has been postponed. Refer to the Imaging Efficiency Measures for more information.

[b] OP-19 has been removed; however, submission of a "nonblank" value is required through Q4 2013 encounters.

Adapted from QualityNet. Hospital outpatient quality reporting program. Available at: http://www.qualitynet.org/dcs/ContentServer?cid=1192804531207&pagename=QnetPublic%2FPage%2FQnetTier3&c=Page. Accessed July 14, 2015.

Local Measures to Demonstrate Local Value Improvement

The specific performance measures used as value targets were percentage of on-time starts, operations past 5 PM, average turnover time, average staff overtime, and operating rooms saved. In addition, the financial performance metric was a normalized average daily financial yield adjusted for fixed (daily operational cost) and variable (overtime) personnel costs. To achieve these value measures, additional, intermediate measures were used to track important processes. For instance, patient wait times at the surgical admissions desk and on-time arrival (within 30 minutes of scheduled report time) to the preoperative area were tracked, and both improved favorably. Other specific process improvements included substantial improvements in on-time starts, reductions in the number of cases going past 5 PM, and substantial reductions in nonoperative time, staff overtime, and operating rooms saved. Finally, an efficiency measure of adjusted financial margin per operating room per day demonstrated improvement.

Demonstrating Value May Be More Difficult than Delivering Value

The above example was undertaken in a multispecialty group practice with case volumes exceeding 50,000 cases per year. The approach to process improvement and tracking of performance measures was resource intensive. In all, this approach may not be applicable to other settings. The example of creating local measures to demonstrate value holds, however, and may be applicable in simplified terms for lower-volume settings or hospitals in which stakeholders are not part of a multispecialty group practice.

SUMMARY

When attempting to achieve high-value care for patients, performance measures may play the role of distractor or they may focus efforts to align goals of care among diverse stakeholders. If anesthesiologists wish to demonstrate the value of the care they provide, they should consider the audience for whom they are demonstrating value and the strengths and weaknesses of different measure types. Stronger links between performance measures and payment, in particular by CMS, motivate anesthesiologists to take notice of externally reported performance measures. Such measures may be inferior to locally derived measures when attempting to drive and demonstrate efficiency as a value target.

ACKNOWLEDGMENTS

The authors thank Michael A. Kelm, MD, of Madison Anesthesiology Consultants for thoughtful commentary on the article.

REFERENCES

1. Donabedian A. Evaluating the quality of medical care. 1966. Milbank Q 2005; 83(4):691–729.
2. Brook RH. The end of the quality improvement movement: long live improving value. JAMA 2010;304(16):1831–2.
3. Available at: qualityforum.org. Accessed February 20, 2015.
4. Berry SA, Doll MC, McKinley KE, et al. ProvenCare: quality improvement model for designing highly reliable care in cardiac surgery. Qual Saf Health Care 2009;18(5):360–8.
5. Casale AS, Paulus RA, Selna MJ, et al. "ProvenCareSM": a provider-driven pay-for-performance program for acute episodic cardiac surgical care. Ann Surg 2007;246(4):613–21 [discussion: 621–3].

6. Hyder JA, Hirschberg RE, Nguyen LL. Home discharge as a performance metric for surgery. JAMA Surg 2015;150(2):96–7.
7. Haynes AB, Weiser TG, Berry WR, et al. A surgical safety checklist to reduce morbidity and mortality in a global population. N Engl J Med 2009; 360(5):491–9.
8. Urbach DR, Govindarajan A, Saskin R, et al. Introduction of surgical safety checklists in Ontario, Canada. N Engl J Med 2014;370(11):1029–38.
9. Semel ME, Resch S, Haynes AB, et al. Adopting a surgical safety checklist could save money and improve the quality of care in U.S. hospitals. Health Aff (Millwood) 2010;29(9):1593–9.
10. Gawande AA. 2015. Available at: http://theincidentaleconomist.com/wordpress/when-checklists-work-and-when-they-dont/. Accessed February 20, 2015.
11. Services CfMaM. Available at: cms.gov. Accessed February 12, 2015.
12. Eappen S, Lane BH, Rosenberg B, et al. Relationship between occurrence of surgical complications and hospital finances. JAMA 2013;309(15):1599–606.
13. Scally CP, Thumma JR, Birkmeyer JD, et al. Impact of surgical quality improvement on payments in medicare patients. Ann Surg 2015;262(2):249–52.
14. Porter ME. What is value in health care? N Engl J Med 2010;363(26):2477–81.
15. Hyder JA, Roy N, Wakeam E, et al. Performance measurement in surgery through the National Quality Forum. J Am Coll Surg 2014;219(5):1037–46.
16. Hyder JA, Niconchuk J, Glance LG, et al. What can the national quality forum tell us about performance measurement in anesthesiology? Anesth Analg 2015; 120(2):440–8.
17. Hoy EW. The surgical CAHPS survey. Bull Am Coll Surg 2009;94(7):6–7.
18. Hyder JA. Pain-free surgery or pain-free parking: measuring patient satisfaction with perioperative care is humbling for the anesthesiologist. Anesthesiology 2014;120(3):780–1.
19. Available at: qualityforum.org. CMS List of Measures under Consideration for December 1, 2014. Accessed February 12, 2015.
20. O'Malley AJ, Zaslavsky AM, Hays RD, et al. Exploratory factor analyses of the CAHPS Hospital Pilot Survey responses across and within medical, surgical, and obstetric services. Health Serv Res 2005;40(6 Pt 2):2078–95.
21. Fiscella K, Burstin HR, Nerenz DR. Quality measures and sociodemographic risk factors: to adjust or not to adjust. JAMA 2014;312(24):2615–6.
22. Lawson EH, Louie R, Zingmond DS, et al. A comparison of clinical registry versus administrative claims data for reporting of 30-day surgical complications. Ann Surg 2012;256(6):973–81.
23. Wakeam E, Hyder JA, Jiang W, et al. Risk and patterns of secondary complications in surgical inpatients. JAMA Surg 2015;150(1):65–73.
24. Bilimoria KY, Chung J, Ju MH, et al. Evaluation of surveillance bias and the validity of the venous thromboembolism quality measure. JAMA 2013;310(14):1482–9.
25. Kinnier CV, Barnard C, Bilimoria KY. The need to revisit VTE quality measures. JAMA 2014;312(3):286–7.
26. Pagel C, Brown KL, Crowe S, et al. A mortality risk model to adjust for case mix in UK paediatric cardiac surgery. Southampton (United Kingdom): NIHR Journals Library, Health Services and Delivery Research; 2013.
27. Maradit Kremers H, Lewallen LW, Lahr BD, et al. Do Claims-based Comorbidities Adequately Capture Case Mix for Surgical Site Infections? Clin Orthop Relat Res 2015;473(5):1777–86.

28. Raval MV, Cohen ME, Ingraham AM, et al. Improving American College of Surgeons National Surgical Quality Improvement Program risk adjustment: incorporation of a novel procedure risk score. J Am Coll Surg 2010;211(6):715–23.
29. Krell RW, Hozain A, Kao LS, et al. Reliability of risk-adjusted outcomes for profiling hospital surgical quality. JAMA Surg 2014;149(5):467–74.
30. Lawson EH, Ko CY, Adams JL, et al. Reliability of evaluating hospital quality by colorectal surgical site infection type. Ann Surg 2013;258(6):994–1000.
31. Frank SM, Fleisher LA, Breslow MJ, et al. Perioperative maintenance of normothermia reduces the incidence of morbid cardiac events. A randomized clinical trial. JAMA 1997;277(14):1127–34.
32. Ingraham AM, Cohen ME, Bilimoria KY, et al. Association of surgical care improvement project infection-related process measure compliance with risk-adjusted outcomes: implications for quality measurement. J Am Coll Surg 2010;211(6):705–14.
33. Shih T, Dimick JB. Reliability of readmission rates as a hospital quality measure in cardiac surgery. Ann Thorac Surg 2014;97(4):1214–8.
34. Gonzalez AA, Girotti ME, Shih T, et al. Reliability of hospital readmission rates in vascular surgery. J Vasc Surg 2014;59(6):1638–43.
35. Tsai TC, Orav EJ, Jha AK. Care fragmentation in the postdischarge period: surgical readmissions, distance of travel, and postoperative mortality. JAMA Surg 2015;150(1):59–64.
36. Gonzalez AA, Shih T, Dimick JB, et al. Using same-hospital readmission rates to estimate all-hospital readmission rates. J Am Coll Surg 2014;219(4):656–63.
37. www.sts.org. Available at: http://www.sts.org/sts-national-database/adult-cardiac-anesthesia-module. Accessed February 20, 2015.
38. Etzioni DA, Wasif N, Dueck AC, et al. Association of hospital participation in a surgical outcomes monitoring program with inpatient complications and mortality. JAMA 2015;313(5):505–11.
39. Osborne NH, Nicholas LH, Ryan AM, et al. Association of hospital participation in a quality reporting program with surgical outcomes and expenditures for Medicare beneficiaries. JAMA 2015;313(5):496–504.
40. Kazaure HS, Martin M, Yoon JK, et al. Long-term results of a postoperative pneumonia prevention program for the inpatient surgical ward. JAMA Surg 2014;149(9):914–8.
41. Cima R, Dankbar E, Lovely J, et al. Colorectal surgery surgical site infection reduction program: a national surgical quality improvement program–driven multidisciplinary single-institution experience. J Am Coll Surg 2013;216(1):23–33.
42. Cima RR, Lackore KA, Nehring SA, et al. How best to measure surgical quality? Comparison of the Agency for Healthcare Research and Quality Patient Safety Indicators (AHRQ-PSI) and the American College of Surgeons National Surgical Quality Improvement Program (ACS-NSQIP) postoperative adverse events at a single institution. Surgery 2011;150(5):943–9.
43. Hashmi ZG, Dimick JB, Efron DT, et al. Reliability adjustment: a necessity for trauma center ranking and benchmarking. J Trauma Acute Care Surg 2013;75(1):166–72.
44. Cohen ME, Ko CY, Bilimoria KY, et al. Optimizing ACS NSQIP modeling for evaluation of surgical quality and risk: patient risk adjustment, procedure mix adjustment, shrinkage adjustment, and surgical focus. J Am Coll Surg 2013;217(2):336–46.e1.
45. Salkowski N, Snyder JJ, Zaun DA, et al. Bayesian methods for assessing transplant program performance. Am J Transpl 2014;14(6):1271–6.

46. Henneman D, van Bommel AC, Snijders A, et al. Ranking and rankability of hospital postoperative mortality rates in colorectal cancer surgery. Ann Surg 2014;259(5):844–9.

47. Merkow RP, Ju MH, Chung JW, et al. Underlying reasons associated with hospital readmission following surgery in the United States. JAMA 2015;313(5):483–95.

48. Larson DW, Lovely JK, Cima RR, et al. Outcomes after implementation of a multimodal standard care pathway for laparoscopic colorectal surgery. Br J Surg 2014;101(8):1023–30.

49. Lee TH. Eulogy for a quality measure. N Engl J Med 2007;357(12):1175–7.

50. Stain SC, Hoyt DB, Hunter JG, et al. American surgery and the Affordable Care Act. JAMA Surg 2014;149(9):984–5.

51. DeJohn P. New quality measures, tight deadline mark CMS payment rule for ASCs. OR Manager 2013;29(10):28–30.

52. Available at: www.aamc.org. Accessed February 12, 2015.

53. Available at: www.aha.org. Accessed February 20, 2015.

54. www.asahq.org. Available at: http://www.asahq.org/resources/quality-improvement/qcdr/available-measures. Accessed February 18, 2015.

55. Centers for Medicare & Medicaid Services (CMS), HHS. Medicare and Medicaid programs: hospital outpatient prospective payment and ambulatory surgical center payment systems and quality reporting programs; Hospital Value-Based Purchasing Program; organ procurement organizations; quality improvement organizations; Electronic Health Records (EHR) Incentive Program; provider reimbursement determinations and appeals. Final rule with comment period and final rules. Fed Regist 2013;78(237):74825–5200.

56. Cima RR, Brown MJ, Hebl JR, et al. Use of lean and six sigma methodology to improve operating room efficiency in a high-volume tertiary-care academic medical center. J Am Coll Surg 2011;213(1):83–92 [discussion: 93–4].

Optimizing Operating Room Scheduling

Wilton C. Levine, MD, Peter F. Dunn, MD*

KEYWORDS

- Operating room schedule • Operating room resource management
- Operating room design • OR case length • OR case order
- Post anesthesia care unit (PACU) flow

KEY POINTS

- The operating room (OR) schedule is a powerful tool to facilitate hospital-wide communication and staffing.
- A well-coordinated schedule can significantly impact patient throughput through the entire hospital.
- The OR schedule provides a wealth of data that should be used for appropriate resource planning.
- Governance and management of the OR schedule impacts OR success, including patient safety and productivity.

The operating room (OR) schedule is a living and breathing organism filled with patients needing elective, urgent, and emergent operations. When considering how to increase surgical volume and patient access, there are often 2 main strategies: build additional surgical suites or improve surgical efficiency. The former takes significant time, planning, and financial resources and the latter takes strong leadership and organizational planning with an effective OR team.[1] Effective organization and management of the OR schedule is critical to ensure ready access for all patient types within your organization and appropriate operating time for surgeons, while simultaneously ensuring the success of your OR, surgical practices, the hospital and health care.

In this article, we review the essential elements of OR schedule management. We discuss the use of the OR as a resource to ensure efficient patient access and organizational efficiency, and discuss methods that can be applied to add value to your

Drs P.F. Dunn and W.C. Levine do not have any commercial or financial conflicts of interest or any funding related to the ideas or material discussed in this article.
Perioperative Services, Massachusetts General Hospital, 55 Fruit Street, White 400, Boston, MA 02114, USA
* Corresponding author.
E-mail address: pdunn@partners.org

organization through optimal OR schedule management. In doing so, we discuss methods to create an OR schedule, its use for resource planning before the day of surgery and as a dynamic roadmap intraday not only for the flow of patients in the perioperative environment but throughout the hospital as well. The OR schedule is a tool not only to help manage patient flow, but also the flow of other hospital resources, such as equipment, instrumentation, and ancillary hospital staffing resources. The OR schedule generates a vast dataset that may be used for future planning and process improvement. Through our discussion, we review some basic definitions, global block schedule management, block allocation and block release, daily schedule management, OR patient flow, and the impact of post anesthesia care unit (PACU) management on the OR schedule.

Definitions

Surgical block: Specific OR(s) and time(s) where designated surgeons or surgical services perform their surgical cases.

Block schedule: The schedule of ORs and associated times assigned to surgeons and/or surgical service (**Fig. 1**).

Surgeon-specific block: A surgical block assigned to a specific surgeon.

Service-specific block: A surgical block assigned to a specific surgical service, practice, or group of surgeons.

Open block: A surgical block without specific surgeon assignment. Typically, this is a surgical block held for add-on cases.

Block release: The methodology for finalization of the OR schedule describing how far in advance cases may be freely added and when the OR schedule is considered closed.

Scheduled case: A surgical case known and planned in advance of the day of surgery. The patient may either come from home or start as an in-patient in the hospital.

Add-on case: A surgical case not known to the OR before the day of surgery. These surgical cases may be nonurgent, urgent, or emergent.

Nonurgent case: An add-on surgical case that needs to be completed within a day of scheduling.

Urgent case: An add-on surgical case that needs to be completed within a predetermined time period because of medical needs. This may be defined as anywhere between 2 and 6 hours depending on the institution and sometimes is broken into subclassifications.

Emergent case: An add-on surgical case that must be performed immediately because of life-threatening medical needs.

Anesthesiologist-in-charge or staff administrator: Senior anesthesiologist managing the intraday flow of cases and resources in the OR in partnership with a senior resource nurse.

BLOCK SCHEDULE MANAGEMENT

Typically, the OR schedule is composed of various types of surgical block allocations known as "block time." Although block time is ultimately an institutional resource, it is often designated for specific surgeons, practices, or patient types. Block time may be assigned based on historic case volume, anticipated case volume, OR utilization reviews, or other criteria. OR leaders work to match elective cases and OR staffing through the use of OR block time in an effort to maximize OR utilization.[2] A common OR block schedule schema includes surgeon-specific block time, service-specific block time, and open block time. Depending on the institutional size and needs, open block time may be fully flexible and designated for all patient and case types,

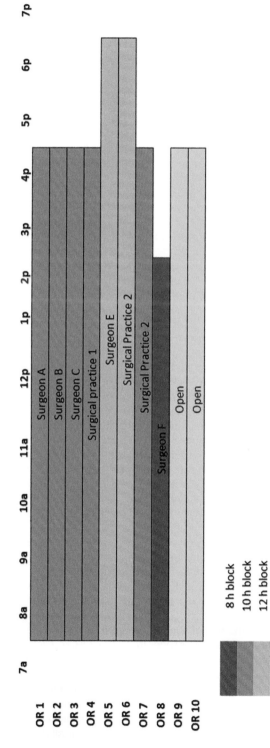

Example Surgical Block Schedule

Fig. 1. A generic surgical block schedule. Patterns may repeat daily, weekly, monthly, or as required by the institutional practice.

may have limited flexibility specifically oriented for particular patient and case types, or may be nonflexible and designated specifically for a singular type of case.[3–5]

Surgeon-specific blocks are allocated by an institution for primary use by an individual surgeon. These blocks may recur weekly, monthly, or in some other recursive pattern. Surgeon-specific blocks allow a surgeon to coordinate a regular schedule for surgery, clinic, and other related activities.

Service-specific blocks are allocated by an institution for primary use by a group of surgeons, practice, or surgical service. This type of block allocation may allow for service-specific add-on cases and OR time for surgeons needing operative time above their standard surgeon-specific blocks. Service-specific blocks are also effective for surgical practices that function as a group practice rather than individual practices. For example, this is increasingly found with orthopedic trauma and general trauma services at tertiary care hospitals.[6]

A split block is a full surgical block divided into 2 or more smaller surgical blocks within a single day. Use of split blocks requires highly predictable OR case length with little risk of cases running past the end of the scheduled time.[7] These blocks are often effective in ambulatory surgical centers and small hospitals. In our experience, they are less effective in academic medical centers and trauma centers.

Open blocks are allocated by an institution to be staffed in anticipation of cases to be added on the day of surgery. This openness allows for the timely placement of add-on surgical cases without the disruption of the scheduled surgical cases. A mix of scheduled case volume, add-on case volume and surgeon availability are some of the key, data-driven metrics that each institution needs to consider when deciding how to allocate the OR resources in this manner for the proper care of their patients.[4]

Once the block schedule is determined, appropriate nursing, anesthesia, and support staffing plans can be generated.[8] The block allocation for different services may not be consistent each day of the week and different nursing and anesthesia resources may be required. In addition, an OR may not run the same total number of ORs each day of the week, impacting staffing patterns. Such a variable OR volume may help to smooth out the use of other resources, and, in the end, provide more predictable, timely access to care for all patients.[9]

The effective use of the allocated surgical blocks is critical for the success of the OR. When the blocks are filled predictably with surgical cases, management of staffing resources is straightforward and predictable. However, specific surgeons are not available to fill their blocks across the entire calendar year. Surgeons attend meetings, take vacations, and have other reasons to be away from the OR. As such, communication by the surgeon or practice alerting the OR that they will not be using their surgical block is critical. It is a balance of control and collaboration. How far in advance must a surgeon tell the OR that he or she will not use his block? What are the consequences for failure to communicate this important information? What does the OR administration do with released block time?

To manage staffing effectively, ensure smooth patient care, and have some degree of flexibility, there must be a policy governing how and when surgical blocks will be released in advance of the day of surgery. There are 3 main types of block releases to consider: planned surgeon absence from the OR, preschedule release, and schedule finalization.

Communication on anticipated block usage is critical and blocks should be released when surgeons know they will not use their block for any reason. To be effective, this block release must typically occur at least 2 weeks in advance with the understanding that further in advance is more beneficial. This advance notice allows for either other surgeons to add cases into the released blocks or allows the OR to alter staffing patterns to match the case volume. Depending on the season and schedule, OR management may choose to reallocate the bocks to other surgeons and services or to close the blocks entirely. Consideration for block closure is particularly important over holiday and school vacation weeks when there is high demand from all OR staff for vacation time.

Several days to a week before the day of surgery, the block schedule should release to allow additional cases to be added. In a large institution, these blocks may change from surgeon-specific blocks to service-specific blocks. This allows surgeons within similar specialties to easily add cases to the schedule. In smaller hospitals, nursing staff may have competency to perform all cases and case-specific room allocation may not matter, whereas in larger hospitals nurses are often managed within service-specific pods with service-related competency training. In these instances, keeping the right case mix in the right ORs is critical.

Depending on the surgical service, the release time may vary from 1 day to more than 1 week.[10] As the day of surgery approaches, the schedule must close and no longer allow free access to book additional elective cases. This is necessary to finalize staffing, instrumentation, case carts, and other specific day of surgery planning issues. Despite the schedule closing to new cases, additional add-on cases always appear and we maintain flexibility to accommodate our patient's needs.

As an example, consider standard ORs in a hospital. Each of these ORs release from surgeon-specific blocks to service-specific blocks 5 business days before the day of surgery. Two business days before the day of surgery, the schedule closes and any case additions requires the approval of the OR director or designee.

Within the block schedule and block release patterns, hospitals often have significant numbers of add-on cases. ORs must have an appropriate number of open blocks to accommodate these patients. These are staffed ORs that do not have scheduled cases to allow improved access for urgent patient care without disruption of the electively scheduled patients.[5,11,12] The number and organization of these open blocks depends on the number of daily add-on cases. It has been shown that large-scale application of an open block strategy can significantly improve the flow of nonelective surgery patients. In fact, this strategy applied in our institution reduced patient wait time for surgical procedures by 25% simultaneous to a surgical volume increase of 9%. In addition, patient bed days for this patient population decreased by 13%.[4]

The OR schedule helps to predict the anticipated surgical case mix and allows for appropriate planning of required staffing resources for the OR and for the hospital. Typically, we consider the nursing and anesthesia resources but we must not forget the preoperative/PACU nurses, transport personnel, and room turnover personnel. In academic centers, residency work-hour restrictions have caused a decrease in available residents to assist with operative procedures, leading to needs for additional scrub personnel, RN first assists, and other midlevel assistants. Models have been developed to use the OR schedule as a tool to predict future resource needs up to 2 weeks in advance. With this type of tool, the OR schedule becomes a hospital resource not only to manage the OR, but also to manage other hospital resources like pathology, radiology, physical therapy, and other hospital services.[13]

Monitoring and active management of the OR block schedule is required by OR leadership. Regular communication with surgeons on their individual or practice/departmental utilization fosters teamwork within the OR. Monitoring of the utilization is a straightforward operational metric that is necessary for high-level OR management. Standards may be set by OR leadership to determine how blocks are reallocated when underutilized and how services overutilizing surgical time may acquire additional block time.[14-16] Availability and use of this robust data from the OR schedule and other OR metrics eases the processes when making effective block assignment decisions and facilitates the challenging conversations that go along with that process.

DAILY SCHEDULE MANAGEMENT
Operating Room Schedule

The OR schedule is the central system by which the OR is managed by the OR leadership team and can serve as an effective tool to communicate real-time information for the flow of patients and resources to all departments involved with the care of surgical patients. In our institution, the "active" dynamic OR schedule is accessed by only a few leaders managing the OR each day to avoid any errors with case placement or management. The active schedule can be "viewed" by many people in several different formats. The flow of the patient is depicted in a color diagram for each room and each separate OR location in our system (**Fig. 2**). The colors change through manual timestamps entered into the central perioperative nursing record. The process begins at the patient's first entry point into the perioperative system. This continues through the OR with currently 5 different timestamps recorded: (1) patient into the OR, (2). patient ready for surgery, (3) surgery begins, (4) surgery ends, and (5) the patient leaves the OR. Finally, the patient's care is tracked through the various phases of recovery until discharge to home or another bed in the hospital through additional entries into the perioperative record.

This manual data entry has some gaps (eg, no data entries are available between check in ready and entering OR), which present challenges with process improvement efforts aimed at improving on time starts, turnovers, and so on. Real-time tracking systems offer opportunities to track patients and other assets and automatically link that information to the OR schedule.[17,18] We are currently outfitting all of our perioperative areas to begin system-wide patient tracking. The goal of this investment is to enhance data available for our ongoing process improvement efforts aimed at future efforts to further.

Determining Case Length

A commonly discussed challenge among OR managers and perioperative leaders is how to determine the expected case length for a given operation.[19] The goal is to balance the timeliness of care for all patients, thus requiring degrees of both flexibility and predictability, with the need to efficiently utilize costly resources. If one reduces flexibility, the more restrictive scheduling practice results in underutilization of the OR and leads to longer presurgical wait times because one cannot "pack" the schedule for a given surgeon block. On the other hand, too much flexibility may lead to a less predictable schedule on the day of surgery, incur significant overtime costs for staff, and may cause intraday delays leading to day of surgery cancellations.

Multiple studies have examined the problem in great detail and many recommended solutions to this apparent Gordian knot exist.[20,21] The summation of the body of work to date is that no one methodology will fit all OR scheduling challenges, but a systematic approach tailored to one's institution is essential to get to a balanced state of effectiveness. At our institution, we utilize the following components to the methodology for case scheduling. First, surgeons book each case using a homegrown scheduling code. The surgeons are free to add codes that best fit their practices. Second, surgeon-specific historical data for each scheduling code is maintained and the duration of the procedure is booked using the running average of their last 10 cases. The booking case times are for "wheels in" to "wheels out." In instances where a surgeon

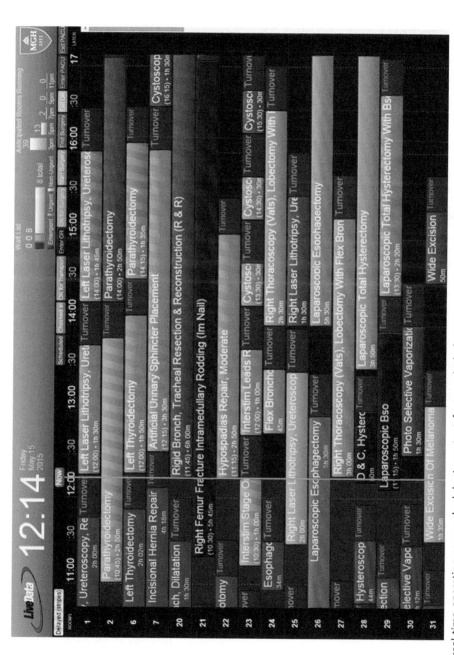

Fig. 2. A real-time operating room schedule. Important features include: current time and date (*upper left*), real-time count of add-on cases and predicted rooms running by hour of day (*upper right*), colors to indicate patient location, case status and case progression (*color grid at top of black section on upper right*).

has no data for a given scheduling code, the service-specific average is used for the surgeon's first case. If no previous case exists at all, an arbitrary value is used (2.5 hours). We monitor the schedule for the inappropriate use of new or unused scheduling codes to shorten established case booking times. Third, the surgeons are allowed to book a case longer than the historical average, but may not shorten the case without a conversation with the staff administrator managing the ORs for the day in question or one of us. We assign an arbitrary, service-specific turnover time assigned to the service of the previous case in instances where the following case is another service. We believe this type of data-driven approach balances the inaccuracies incurred with surgeon prediction alone and the inability of any mathematical methodology to replace clinical intuition.[19]

Despite the application of any type of methodology, intraday issues, and case-specific elements still contribute to variations against some standard. Studying one's own institution and monitoring data is essential for the ongoing tweaking to the system. Such elements as communication, team constituency, and team training are important variables to consider, which may impact the intraday schedule.[22,23]

Case Order

The planning for the timely access to care for all of the surgical patients does not begin on the day of surgery. As mentioned, the global and specific assignment of the blocks, the ongoing assessment of block performance, and the management of those blocks up until the day of surgery are essential tasks for proper management of the OR resources and much work has been done in each of these areas.[2,8,15] Less effort has focused on the intrablock arrangement of the specific order of the cases with an aim toward OR and perioperative system efficiency. Rather, intraday case order studies have focused more on the various clinical issues that may be relevant to particular patients, such as age, diabetes mellitus, timing of dialysis, and coordination with other services such as radiology, pathology, and radiation services, to name a few.[24]

As a typical academic medical center that serves as a community hospital for our local citizens as well as a quaternary referral center for complex procedures, there are many variations to the case volume and complexity to each block each day. They range from single case rooms running for more than 12 hours and involving multiple specialties and many shifts of support staff to a single surgeon room with more than 12 simple, outpatient procedures. The midpoint of that range is an OR with a mix of inpatients and outpatient cases, for both single and multiple surgeons alike. The summary output of those blocks in total and its variability can have a significant impact on the use of the resources throughout the hospital. Our team has modeled and implemented a system-wide block strategy that has had much success in smoothing our bed capacity problem.[25] More recently, we performed a modeling project on the impact of the intrablock case order aimed at further mitigating the congestion we face each day in the perioperative environment and hospital by reordering the case sequence in appropriate blocks.[26]

The data driven model aimed at reducing delays within the perioperative system model had 4 key recommendations. (1) Schedule all patients requiring inpatient beds postoperatively (except for patients already in the same bed preoperatively) as late in the block as possible. (2) Use the finalized planned schedule in advance (24 or 48 hours) to determine the needed discharges by time of day for each floor. (3) Assign beds intraday on a just in time, first come, first serve basis. (4) Enhance process and communication between the PACU and the receiving floor to reduce the handoff time for each patient. Implementing the case resequencing model alone resulted in a 49% reduction in our current perioperative delays for our postoperative patients. This change will not adversely affect the flow of our preoperative patients sharing the same resources. The model also produces a per-floor discharge bed need by hour of day for the next surgical day, allowing for more effective planning and resource management compared with the historical plan of "get everyone out by 1000." Finally, we are modeling currently the transition to a just in time bed assignment with our admitting and floor teams for all inpatient bed assignments. It is believed that this change will result in much improved patient processing times and reduction of delays throughout all areas of the hospital.

POST ANESTHESIA CARE UNIT FLOW

The PACU serves a multitude of functions within an academic medical center. In addition to serving as both preoperative and postoperative patient care functions (thus, we use the term perioperative bay and have built all of our newer spaces as individual standard bays with centralized support functions; **Fig. 3**), our PACU is also used for ICU care (either planned or as overflow), electroconvulsive therapy, outpatient peripherally inserted central catheter placement, and as a backup for off-hour dialysis care if the dialysis unit is off line. It becomes an easy buffer for offsetting more system-wide congestion problems, which allows for the ongoing performance of the OR without addressing the primary problem. Many studies have indeed looked at the relationship of the operating schedule and the PACU resources, with subsequent

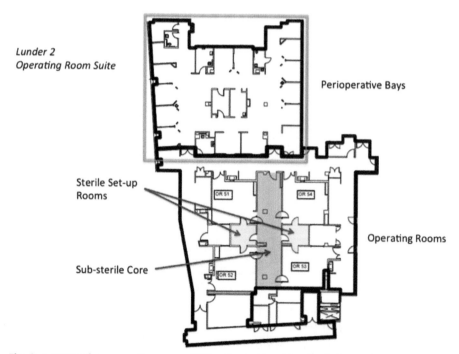

Fig. 3. Layout of an operating room (OR) suite designed for flexibility and patient privacy. Perioperative bays facilitate preoperative and postoperative care. Sterile setup rooms facilitate setup of surgical equipment and rapid OR turnover. (*From* Agarwala A, Levine WC, Germain B, et al. Innovative surgical suite design improves OR efficiency. Presentation at American Society of Anesthesiologists Annual Meeting. October 15, 2013. San Francisco, California; with permission.)

recommendations aimed at optimizing patient perioperative throughput.[27] In 2009, we published the findings from our own study performed in the planning stages of a new building with 28 additional ORs and an unplanned number of perioperative bays.[28] We did know that surgical services would not have an increase in the inpatient bed capacity coupled with the new ORs. In this study, we assessed the variable impact of and the sensitive relationship between the OR case load, the number of recovery beds, and the magnitude of recovery congestion. The relationship is depicted in **Fig. 4** and allows one to understand the impact of one variable on the others. We used this model to help drive and support the number of perioperative bays in our new building.

Subsequent work revealed that the PACU should not be the endpoint of the OR–PACU congestion story. In subsequent works, we have shown that the OR schedule and primarily the elective case volume being admitted to the hospital after surgery is the primary driver of the congestion. However, the congestion lies not in the PACU, but in the floor beds. As shown in **Fig. 5**, the typical midweek and midday congestion is driven most by the elective surgical population with hospital lengths of stay fewer than 7 days. We constructed an optimization model to find a rearrangement of the elective block schedule to smooth out the average inpatient census by reducing the maximum average occupancy throughout the week. Approximately 21% of all blocks were rearranged and the end result was a decrease in the peak census by 3.2% while allowing for a 9% growth in surgical volume over the study period. In addition, the delays occurring between the OR and the PACU decreased

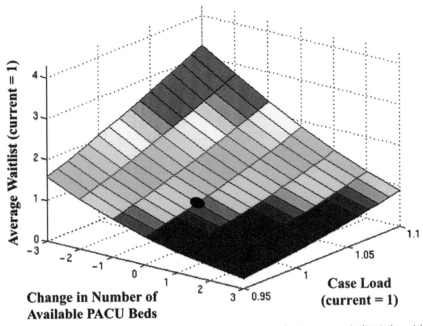

Fig. 4. Three-dimensional surface of cumulative post anesthesia care unit (PACU) waitlist time as a function of PACU capacity and operating room caseload. Current state is identified by the black dot. Functional PACU capacity is limited to 24 beds. This gives an average weekly cumulative PACU waitlist of about 21 patient-hours in the current state. (*From* Schoenmeyr T, Dunn PF, Gamarnik D, et al. A model for understanding the impacts of demand and capacity on waiting time to enter a congested recovery room. Anesthesiology 2009;110(6):1303; with permission.)

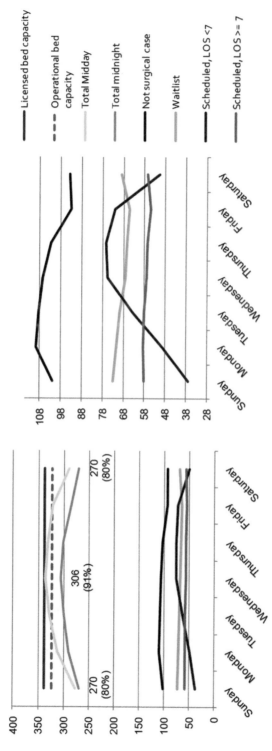

Fig. 5. Average midnight census in the surgical wards. LOS, length of stay.

from a daily and monthly average of 19% of the total case volume experiencing delays before implementation of the schedule changes to fewer than 5% since the changes to present day.

Few institutions have the luxury of creating additional PACU capacity to buffer their OR efficiency against hospital-wide congestion. In addition to considering major changes as noted, which require significant institutional leadership support and operations research resources, OR leaders can drive operational changes within their own environment to bring about beneficial effects.

Similar to other academic medical centers, we have many different patient types flowing through the same system. Unlike dedicated ambulatory surgical centers, where the entire team is trained to care for a uniform, outpatient case mix, our perioperative teams face the challenges of those same efficiency needs for our outpatients alongside some of the most complex, resource and time intensive patients. This is a dilemma that could most easily be solved by physically separating the 2 disparate patient streams through the entire perioperative process. However, for us, and we suspect most other academic medical centers, this not a viable solution without some additional, major investment in building and staffing resources.

We did learn through patient flow simulation efforts that our 1-size fits all method of a multiphase recovery in multiple locations was contributing immensely to the inefficiencies we faced.[29] The model determined that we could recover many of our outpatients in a 1 phase, single location without adversely affecting care for those patients or others. In addition, many of our teams were doing this already in a "reactive" mode when there were delays transferring from the first recovery area to the discharge recovery space. The modeled showed that implementing a 1-stage recovery process proactively for outpatients was feasible and would reduce the PACU congestion by 27%. Implementing such process changes based on data-driven models is an important tool for OR leaders to use when facing such capacity challenges.[30,31]

Additional Considerations

For high-volume surgeons, the goal of OR scheduling is to provide a system within which the perioperative team is able to support efficient, high-quality care to each patient. As mentioned, academic medical centers have many types of patients and surgery practices to accommodate, so a singular process does not support all patients adequately. Previous work has shown that parallel processing and facility design can have major impact on providing nodes of high efficiency within the perioperative suite.[32] Beyond the 1-room model in the study of Sandberg and colleagues[33] we have shown in subsequent work that an entire OR suite designed specifically for high-volume, rapid turnover can further advance the efficiency of a highly performing OR team (see Fig. 4). The key elements in that design are the high ratio of perioperative bays to ORs (13:4), instrument setup rooms between each OR pair, and clinician work stations within the suite. Using this design, the efficiency gain for high-volume surgeons has resulted in additional cases per day, thus providing more timely access to care for many patients.

Another way to accommodate high-volume surgeons is to assign parallel blocks on his or her surgery day, often called concurrent surgery. Critics may argue that such practices could result in less efficient use of overall perioperative resources for the sake of surgeon efficiency. To be sure, ongoing monitoring of the surgical outcomes and the proper use of perioperative resources is necessary for patient safety and cost effectiveness, respectively. Careful planning of the intraday case management by the surgeon and the team is critical to ensure compliance with national regulations for billing are met as well. When properly performed, concurrent surgery yields favorable outcomes for the system and patients.[34] In addition to the increased timely access to care such parallel processing affords patients, it is also an essential component in academic medical centers for the graduated responsibility of our trainees.[35]

SUMMARY

Whether you work in an academic medical center or ambulatory surgical center, the OR schedule is an important tool generating vast and significant data. The OR schedule allows staff in the OR and hospital from surgeons, anesthesiologists, nurses, technicians, and ancillary staff along with other hospital based departments to plan resources and appropriately allocate staff. Data-driven schedule management allows improved use of hospital resources and may decrease hospital occupancy through matched allocation of operative procedures across the week. Similarly, case booking time and case order impact the daily flow of patients throughout the day and must be considered during the schedule preparation. The PACU is an important buffer within the hospital for preoperative patients, postoperative patients, and sometimes for ICU and other patient types. Most important, the OR schedule provides a platform for coordinated leadership and governance to ensure smooth comprehensive management from the strategic block schedule through to the daily management in the OR and PACU and beyond.

REFERENCES

1. Price DJ. Managing variability to improve quality, capacity and cost in the perioperative process at Massachusetts General Hospital, in MIT Sloan School of Management and the Engineering Systems Division. Cambridge (MA): Massachusetts Institute of Technology; 2011. p. 42.
2. Dexter F, Macario A, Traub RD, et al. An operating room scheduling strategy to maximize the use of operating room block time: computer simulation of patient scheduling and survey of patients' preferences for surgical waiting time. Anesth Analg 1999;89(1):7–20.
3. Zonderland ME, Boucherie RJ, Litvak N, et al. Planning and scheduling of semi-urgent surgeries. Health Care Manag Sci 2010;13(3):256–67.
4. Zenteno A, Carnes T, Levi R, et al. Pooled open blocks shorten wait times for nonelective surgical cases. Ann Surg 2015;262(1):60–7.
5. Ferrand YB, Magazine MJ, Rao US. Partially flexible operating rooms for elective and emergency surgeries. Decis Sci J 2014;45(5):819–47.
6. Bhattacharyya T, Vrahas MS, Morrison SM, et al. The value of the dedicated orthopaedic trauma operating room. J Trauma 2006;60(6):1336–40 [discussion: 1340–1].
7. Patterson P. A few simple rules for managing block time in the operating room. OR Manager 2004;20(11):1–7.
8. McIntosh C, Dexter F, Epstein RH. The impact of service-specific staffing, case scheduling, turnovers, and first-case starts on anesthesia group and operating room productivity: a tutorial using data from an Australian hospital. Anesth Analg 2006;103(6):1499–516.
9. Dunn PF, Levi R. Systematic block allocation in academic medical centers. 2013 DIIE collaborative academic/practitioner workshop on operational innovation. London: London Business School, Regent's Park; 2013.
10. Mazzei WJ. 25 years and 150 medical centers. 2015. Available at: http://perioperativesummit.org/uploads/3/2/2/1/3221254/1_mazzei_friday_am_-or_workshop_2015.pdf. Accessed May 1, 2015.

11. Heng M, Wright JG. Dedicated operating room for emergency surgery improves access and efficiency. Can J Surg 2013;56(3):167–74.
12. Erdem E, Xiuli Q, Shi J. Rescheduling of elective patients upon the arrival of emergency patients. Decis Support Syst 2012;54:551–63.
13. Tiwari V, Furman WR, Sandberg WS. Predicting case volume from the accumulating elective operating room schedule facilitates staffing improvements. Anesthesiology 2014;121(1):171–83.
14. Dexter F, Macario A, Traub RD, et al. Operating room utilization alone is not an accurate metric for the allocation of operating room block time to individual surgeons with low caseloads. Anesthesiology 2003;98(5):1243–9.
15. Dexter F, Traub RD, Macario A. How to release allocated operating room time to increase efficiency: predicting which surgical service will have the most underutilized operating room time. Anesth Analg 2003;96(2):507–12.
16. Dexter F, Macario A. When to release allocated operating room time to increase operating room efficiency. Anesth Analg 2004;98(3):758–62. table of contents.
17. Egan MT, Sandberg WS. Auto identification technology and its impact on patient safety in the Operating Room of the Future. Surg Innov 2007;14(1):41–50 [discussion: 51].
18. Levine WC, Meyer M, Egan M, et al. Development of a vendor agnostic, full disclosure system for capture, display, and storage of operative systems data. AMIA Annu Symp Proc 2006;1006.
19. Joustra P, Meester R, van Ophem H. Can statisticians beat surgeons at the planning of operations. Empir Econ 2013;2013(44):1697–818.
20. Eijkemans MJ, van Houdenhoven M, Nguyen T, et al. Predicting the unpredictable: a new prediction model for operating room times using individual characteristics and the surgeon's estimate. Anesthesiology 2010;112(1):41–9.
21. Dexter F, Macario A, Ledolter J. Identification of systematic underestimation (bias) of case durations during case scheduling would not markedly reduce overutilized operating room time. J Clin Anesth 2007;19(3):198–203.
22. Gillespie BM, Chaboyer W, Fairweather N. Factors that influence the expected length of operation: results of a prospective study. BMJ Qual Saf 2012;21(1):3–12.
23. Entin EB, Lai F, Barach P. Training teams for the perioperative environment: a research agenda. Surg Innov 2006;13(3):170–8.
24. Levine WC, Massachusetts General Hospital. Department of Anesthesia and Critical Care. Handbook of clinical anesthesia procedures of the Massachusetts General Hospital. 8th edition. Philadelphia: Wolters Kluwer Health/Lippincott Williams & Wilkins; 2010. p. 704, xix.
25. Dunn PF, Levi R. Systematic OR block allocation in large academic medical centers. Ann Surg, in press.
26. Range AR. Improving surgical patient flow through simulation of scheduling heuristics, in Massachusetts Institute of Technology Sloan School of Management and the Engineering Systems Division. Cambridge (MA): Massachusetts Institute of Technology; 2013.
27. Marcon E, Dexter F. An observational study of surgeons' sequencing of cases and its impact on postanesthesia care unit and holding area staffing requirements at hospitals. Anesth Analg 2007;105(1):119–26.
28. Schoenmeyr T, Dunn PF, Gamarnik D, et al. A model for understanding the impacts of demand and capacity on waiting time to enter a congested recovery room. Anesthesiology 2009;110(6):1293–304.
29. Schwartz TA. Improving surgical patient flow in a congested recovery area, in Massachusetts Institute of Technology Sloan School of Management and the

Mechanical Engineering Department. Cambridge (MA): Massachusetts Institute of Technology; 2012.

30. Reid PP, Compton WD, Grossman JH, et al. Building a better delivery system: a new engineering/health care partnership. Washington, DC: National Academies Press; 2005.

31. Guerriero F, Guido R. Operational research in the management of the operating theatre: a survey. Health Care Manag Sci 2011;14(1):89–114.

32. Sandberg WS, Daily B, Egan M, et al. Deliberate perioperative systems design improves operating room throughput. Anesthesiology 2005;103(2):406–18.

33. Agarwala A, Levine WC, Germain B, et al. Innovative surgical suite design improves OR efficiency. Presentation at American Society of Anesthesiologists Annual Meeting, October 15, 2013. San Francisco, California.

34. Yount KW, Gillen JR, Kron KL, et al. Attendings' performing simultaneous operations in Academic Cardiothoracic Surgery does not increase operative duration or negatively affect patient outcomes. Paper presented at AATS Annual Meeting. Seattle, WA, April 25–29, 2015. Available at: http://aats.org/annualmeeting/Program-Books/2014/2.cgi. Accessed May 2, 2015.

35. Beasley GM, Pappas TN, Kirk AD. Procedure delegation by attending surgeons performing concurrent operations in academic medical centers: balancing safety and efficiency. Ann Surg 2015;261(6):1044–5.

Lean Strategies in the Operating Room

Stephen T. Robinson, MD, Jeffrey R. Kirsch, MD*

KEYWORDS

- 5S • Just in time production • Leader standard work • Lean management
- Level loading • Standard work • Waste

KEY POINTS

- Lean management strategies can be successfully applied to hospital and operating room environments. It requires management to be fully committed to and actively practice lean management strategies.
- Lean strategies use the pursuit of eliminating waste from the system to leave only the value-added steps in patient care.
- In lean, the patient is the customer. All providers and supporting workers are valued and their engagement is the foundation of using lean strategies.

INTRODUCTION

Lean management has entered many health care systems.[1,2] The origin of this approach is attributed to the Toyota Production System (TPS), which is still the reference organization for outstanding implementation of this approach to excellence.[3,4] Because lean management has arisen from an industry and culture far different from American health care, it is understandable that there is widespread skepticism of using lean approaches to improving a health care organization. Anyone who has worked in health care has seen an array of improvement processes or quality initiatives come and go. Many of these efforts either fail to achieve their goals or fail to sustain them. If an organization is not truly committed to improving itself, then lean strategies are not likely to be any more effective than previously implemented approaches to improvement. What makes using a lean system unique is that it provides the template to create an environment that is continually improving.[5] Other examples of the many excellent resources on lean in health care include books by Albanese and colleagues[6] and Graban.[7]

Both authors have no conflict of interest associated with the content of this article.
Department of Anesthesiology and Perioperative Medicine, Oregon Health & Science University, 3181 Southwest Sam Jackson Park Road, Mail Code KPV5A, Portland, OR 97239, USA
* Corresponding author.
E-mail address: kirschje@ohsu.edu

Anesthesiology Clin 33 (2015) 713–730
http://dx.doi.org/10.1016/j.anclin.2015.07.010
1932-2275/15/$ – see front matter © 2015 Elsevier Inc. All rights reserved.

anesthesiology.theclinics.com

Lean management may look somewhat different based on the unique differences between industries and even between different organizations. Descriptions of lean can be fairly simple or extraordinarily detailed and complex. Although this article is intended to be generic to the health care industry in general and perioperative processes in particular, it is strongly influenced by how it is evolving at Oregon Health & Science University (OHSU).

The use of the vocabulary associated with the TPS has a number of pitfalls. It can reinforce the "has nothing to do with health care" attitude held by many. Worse, it can create a sense of elitism and divide an organization between those who know lean versus those who do not. This is the antithesis of a lean principle that it is the workers who are the source of the solution. Nevertheless, the implementation of any effective system is enhanced when the vocabulary of that system is understood by all. Respectfully introducing lean terms can help draw in clinicians and help them better understand what lean is all about.

Lean management strategy is characterized by the principles of continuous improvement and respect for people. The tools available for lean management are the same as those available to any organization trying to improve its performance. These include 5S (sort, simplify, sweep, standardize, sustain) for organizing work environments, 6 sigma for eliminating defects, control charts, swim lanes for describing individual roles in an ongoing process, and motion tracking, to name just a few. What makes lean unique is the approach to improvement.

To create a lean environment there needs to be a common vision along with the tools and commitment to implement that vision. The underlying concepts can be described as "Methods," "Management System," and "Mindset" (**Fig. 1**).[8] Each is important if lean is going to be successful. There is often conversation regarding whether understanding lean needs to come first or whether doing lean leads to understanding. Different organizations may have different optimal approaches to starting the lean journey. Just like the lean process itself, the reality is that it is an iterative process in which better understanding of lean leads to more successful doing and successful (and even not so successful) doing leads to better understanding.

Sharing a common vision helps orient everyone to the "true north" of an organization's mission. This can be depicted as a Lean House that is built with a foundation of principles, pillars of values, and a roof of the core mission of the organization (**Fig. 2**). The same format can be used to depict the implementation of lean starting

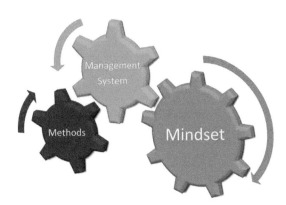

Fig. 1. Three components required to create a lean organization. (*Courtesy of* Joan Wellman & Associates, Inc, ©2015; with permission.)

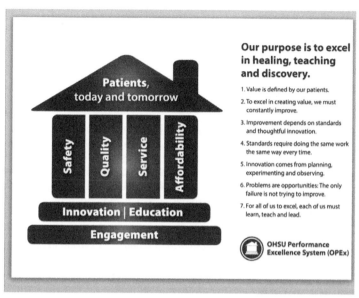

Fig. 2. The OHSU OPEx (lean) House vision statement. (*Courtesy of* Oregon Health & Science University, Portland, OR.)

with a foundation of culture and tools and pillars of lean concepts supporting the goals of the organization (**Fig. 3**).

There are 2 other important core concepts in lean. First, the only customers are the patient and the patient's family. It is designed to focus everyone toward the true north.

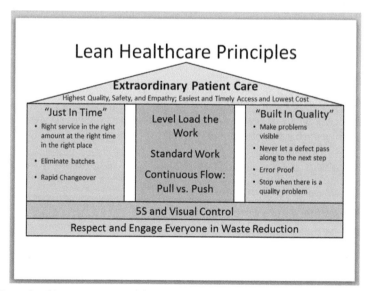

Fig. 3. Example of lean processes used meet organization's mission. Each row may be considered a level to be continuously improved as well as the basis for developing the levels above. (*Courtesy of* Joan Wellman & Associates, Inc, ©2015; with permission.)

It does not diminish the importance of others in the process. As stated previously, lean is built on respect for people. They are simply not customers. The second concept is that lean focuses on problems, not the successes. This does not mean not celebrating or marketing what is done well. It does mean that if an organization wishes to improve, it needs to identify opportunities for improvement and go for it.

LEVEL 1: ENGAGEMENT AND WASTE

The power of lean is that it draws everyone into the improvement process. This can only occur if employees feel secure and respected. This starts with a credible assurance that improving a process will not cause one to lose his or her job. It also requires a belief that one's efforts will actually be considered and perhaps even rewarded. Depending on where an organization is starting, this may come relatively easily or may require a substantial effort from management to demonstrate its sincerity and competence to move forward.

Kaizen is the lean Japanese term for continuous improvement. It emphasizes a team approach to problem solving. It can range from a small group working on a single challenging step of a process to a large, diverse group improving a complex system. The key elements of a Kaizen include stating the problem, objectives, boundaries (in scope and out of scope), core team members, additional resources, and identified leaders. To help focus the effort, this is summarized on a 1-page charter (**Fig. 4**).

SEVEN WASTES

The ideal of lean is to have only value-added steps and eliminate all non–value-added activities that lean identifies as waste. There are commonly 7 identifiable types of

SOR First Case Start Improvement

Problem Statement: Surgeries in SOR have variations in start time regardless of defined 0730/ 0830 Start Times. Since OpTime roll out, three major identified causes of delays: Anesthesia, Systems, and Surgeons. The delays that occur causes variance and delays in the surgery schedule leading to patient, staff and provider dissatisfaction, decreased minutes available for surgical cases, increased non-productive nursing time, increased potential for staff over time, and an inconsistent process that allows opportunity for error.

Goal/Target: Increase on-time starts to >85%.

Objective: Implement a system that includes:
- Standard work for First Case Starts with all stakeholders trained to the Standard Work
- Consistent data monitoring system to evaluate progress or lack of.
- Elimination of waste in workflow for Anesthesia/ PreOp.

In Scope	Out of Scope	Improvement Team
•Patient arrival to 6A • Anesthesia Team: Block/Epidural • 6A Staff •Surgery Team: Surgeon/ SOR •M-F First Case Starts (0830/0730) •Inpatient and Ambulatory Patients	•Weekends • Overnight Stays •Add-on cases (initially only) •ICU direct to OR (initially only)	•Anesthesia Provider •6A Nurse Manager •Performance Improvement Specialist •Surgery Rep •SOR Rep: Circulating RN •6A Workflow Committee

Project Sponsor: Division Director, Periop Services
Process Owner(s): Manager,6A
Facilitators: Performance Improvement Specialist and Nurse Manager

Fig. 4. Problem statement of first case start Kaizen with names deidentified. (*Courtesy of* Oregon Health & Science University, Portland, OR.)

waste (**Table 1**). These are transportation, inventory, motion, waiting, overproduction, overprocessing, and defects. All of these wastes are commonly present in hospitals and operating rooms (ORs). The goal of lean is to have no waste. This may not be completely attainable; however, having the big picture in mind creates an environment in which all waste is on the table and is an opportunity for improvement. Further, the lean process views any reduction of waste as beneficial, and because the emphasis is on continuous improvement, that reduction becomes the new basis for further improvement.

Transportation involves the movement of supplies. Inefficiencies can occur both in the delivery of items to the patient as well as removal of items from the patient. Obtaining medications or blood from a distant pharmacy or blood bank are examples of the former. Getting blood work or pathology specimens to the correct laboratory are examples of the latter. Poor supply planning requiring the transport of supplies to a care area, then moving them back after they are not needed is a common example of this waste.

Reducing transportation waste includes better planning of supply needs and designing better supply flows.

Inventory is an important form of waste. It can be any type of item, such as medications, equipment, or instruments. The most obvious problems with excessive inventory are the capital cost of owning the item and the risk of having expired product; however, excessive inventory can cause additional problems. Changes in usage may make the item obsolete. In addition, the more equipment and supplies in a hospital, the larger the space required to place it. This can make organizing and finding the correct supplies more difficult. It tends to create irregularities in ordering patterns that may lead to not receiving new product when it is actually needed.

Reducing inventory, while ensuring that supplies and equipment are at the right place at the right time, can have a significant impact on value. Implementing just-in-time supply management is an activity that will significantly reduce inventory. To accomplish this objective, rates of use needs to be measured, the supply chain needs

Table 1
The 7 wastes

Waste	Definition	Health Care Examples
Transportation	Unnecessary movement of materials or supplies	Moving samples/specimens, equipment, supplies
Inventory	Supplies, equipment, or information not needed by the customer now	Medications, linens, equipment, parts, supplies, instruments, documents
Motion	Unnecessary movement of people	Moving patients, moving staff, searching for X, getting equipment/supplies
Waiting	Delays in the value stream (absence of flow)	Admission delays, bed assignment delays, testing/treatment delays, discharge delays
Overprocessing	Work that creates no value	Duplication of work, rework, complexity
Overproduction	Producing more than customer needs right now	Treatment or testing done to optimize staff or equipment productivity, not patient needs
Defects/Poor quality	Product or service that does not conform to customer requirements	Medication error, wrong procedure, incorrect X, missing Y, incomplete Z

to be organized and reliable, and the ordering system needs to be simple, reliable, and robust.

Motion is the unnecessary movement of people; both staff and patents. Patients may be asked to travel substantial distances within the hospital to get their needed services. A preoperative visit may involve starting in the parking lot, then on to admitting, the clinic, radiology, blood draw, and back to clinic; or staff may use a substantial amount of time gathering supplies from a wide array of locations. Better organization of a workspace can significantly reduce the distance traveled by a provider (**Fig. 5**).

There are many opportunities to reduce motion. Some can be implemented at the operational level. For patients, valet parking can be offered. Providing more services at the same site is another potential change. For example, have the blood drawn at the clinic. Longer-term solutions may include redesigning the space such that the

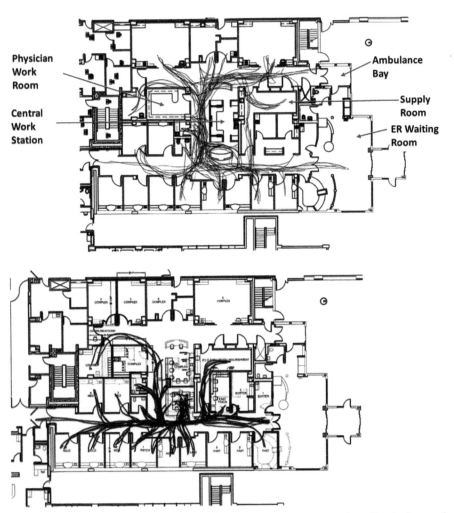

Fig. 5. Actual tracing, spaghetti diagram, of an emergency room nurse's motion before and after a lean improvement project. (*Courtesy of* Joan Wellman & Associates, Inc, ©2015; with permission.)

distance between 2 sites is reduced. For workers, better organization of flow can substantially reduce motion. This is likely to include optimal location of required destinations, such as supplies and pharmaceuticals, and optimal routing to those destinations.

Waiting is a common sight in medical facilities. Like motion, it affects both patients and clinicians. Patients often wait to be seen for their appointments, for expected services, like x-rays or blood draws, at the time of admission and throughout their journey on the day of surgery. Clinicians wait for patients, equipment, supplies, and each other.

Interventions that can limit waiting for patients include more accurate scheduling and reducing the number of steps in the care process. For example, waiting can be reduced if laboratory samples can be drawn at the site of a preoperative visit, rather than needing to go a second location (motion) and then waiting for one's turn.

Overproduction is when more product is made than is needed at that time. It creates inventory that often needs to be transported and stored until it is needed or too often discarded as unnecessary. One example of overproduction is intravenous (IV) setups. Once an IV bag is spiked it has a finite time before it is considered contaminated and must be discarded.

Overproduction can be reduced by limiting the quantities of prepared supplies to those that are known to be needed. Successfully accomplishing this requires a reliable just-in-time process.

Overprocessing is a common source of waste. It includes ordering tests that will not alter patient care. Examples may also include monitoring choices that are not necessary, preparing an array of medication syringes that have little likelihood of being needed (**Fig. 6**), prematurely ordering blood products in low-risk scenarios, preparing multiple endotracheal tubes, or routinely placing a stylet in every endotracheal tube.

In all of these areas, it appears that the culture of being prepared has morphed into being overprepared. The best approach to addressing overprocessing is setting standards that are appropriate to safe patient care. Having reliable delivery of needed supplies and equipment provides greater opportunities to reduce overprocessing. For example, if the blood bank has a reliable turnaround time, then the threshold for requesting blood products can be higher, or if resuscitation syringes can be easily procured, then anesthesia providers in every room will not feel the need to stockpile them.

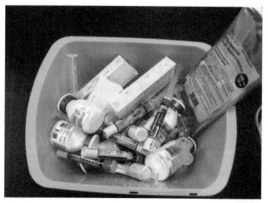

Fig. 6. One of many buckets containing unused syringes and vials collected at the end of the day.

Defects are a critical form of waste. A defect can be identified anywhere from immediately after the time it occurs, to long after the time of the defect. In products, this can cause the need to discard the product, rework the product to eliminate the defect, or dealing with the consequences of having a product returned and the associated need to satisfy a dissatisfied and possibly harmed recipient of the product. Failure to properly sterilize equipment, providing surgical trays with missing or incorrect supplies, and incorrectly assembled pressure transducers are all examples of defects. When adding patients to the formula, the stakes go way up. The quantity and cost of medical errors is well established. In 1999, the Institutes of Medicine estimated that there were 44,000 to 98,000 annual deaths with an associated cost of $17 to $29 billion from increased medical costs and associated lost income and household productivity.[9]

Generally, if a defect can be identified earlier in the process, it will cause less harm and waste. Ignoring defects and waiting for someone else to fix them not only inflates the harm caused by the defect, but increases the likelihood that the same defect will continue to occur. Steps to prevent errors from advancing through the system include empowering workers to identify errors and having processes in place to manage the error once it has been identified. Inspections are important but in lean systems they are really a backstop. The best approach to managing defects is to prevent them in the first place. The more standard the process of producing a product or caring for a patient, the less likely a mistake will be made. The gold standard for preventing defects is error proofing. This involves a system that does not permit a mistake to be made. A simple example of error proofing is the pin index system for gasses. It is (nearly) impossible to misconnect an oxygen delivery system to a nonoxygen gas supply. The joint project to eliminate small-bore tubing misconnects by the Association for the Advancement of Medical Instrumentation and International Organization for Standardization is another. Error proofing may not always be easy, but it has significant potential to reduce harm.[10,11]

LEVEL 2: 5S AND VISUAL CONTROLS

The next level of lean implementation focuses on some of the core tools needed to achieve improvement. The 5S is a stepwise process for organizing a workplace. The steps are sort, simplify, sweep, standardize, and sustain (**Fig. 7**). Having an organized workplace facilitates the effort to reduce waste. It leads to improvements in all forms of waste. It directly reduces transportation, inventory, motion, waiting, and defects while enabling the reduction of overprocessing and overproduction (**Figs. 8** and **9**).

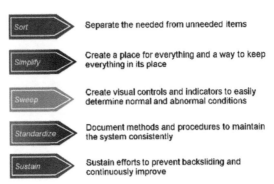

Fig. 7. The 5S process. (*Courtesy of* Joan Wellman & Associates, Inc, ©2015; with permission.)

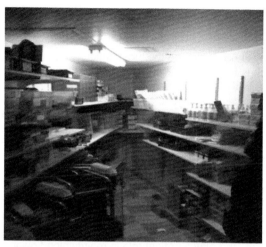

Fig. 8. Supply room before 5S with clutter, nonstandardized, nonvisual, and safety risks. (*Courtesy of* Oregon Health & Science University, Portland, OR.)

Each step has its own intrinsic value as well as being a platform for the next step. Sort separates the needed from the unneeded. One keeps the needed items in a safe, presentable condition. Unneeded items are redeployed where needed, surplused, recycled, or trashed. Simplify is a process that creates a place for everything and a method to keep it in its place. Items are located in a manner that considers safety, effectiveness, and efficiency. For example, frequently used items may be kept closer to the location where they are used. It is an opportunity to determine appropriate quantities of equipment and supplies. Visual outlines and labeling can help ensure that items stay in their correct location.

Sweep (also referred to as shine) is the process in which visual controls are used to identify whether an item is in an acceptable or unacceptable state. This can be identification of items that are above or below minimum levels or items that are ready or not ready for use.

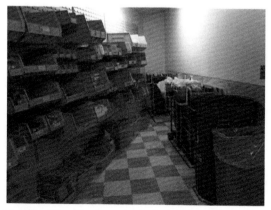

Fig. 9. Supply Room after 5S with clean, logical, visual, and maintainable organization. (*Courtesy of* Oregon Health & Science University, Portland, OR.)

Standardize is a key step that facilitates replicating the 5S process across other work areas. It allows for common practices and methods to be used throughout the affected areas.

Sustain is the key to 5S. It may be the most difficult step, but it is perhaps the hallmark of lean, which is to take every improvement and make it the new normal from which to engage in further improvements. It requires ensuring that everyone understands the new practices and avoids going back to the old ways when things get tough. This is accomplished by visible, ongoing activities that measure and review the status of the workplace (**Fig. 10**). It is also true that optimal results typically take multiple efforts to build on the previous efforts. Each component of 5S has a sequence of levels that identify where in the lean process that step is currently functioning (**Table 2**).

Associated with the 5S process is the emphasis on visual controls. It is often true that one picture is worth a thousand words. They can provide clarity and transparency. The lean term kanban (visual card) is used to describe visual signals (**Fig. 11**). They are associated with inventory control or as part of the process for prominently displaying an identified problem, and play a critical role in maintaining flow in a system.

Visual controls are also used to provide concise communications as well as a record of important information (**Fig. 12**). One example is the use of MESS (materials, equipment, supplies, and staff) to communicate concerns that have been identified early in the day. For example, at OHSU, the inpatient service has a 10-minute gathering that includes representatives supporting services, such as patient transportation, facilities, and purchasing. Problems are quickly identified, countermeasures put in place, and issues needing further work are assigned on the spot (**Fig. 13**). Near the end of the day a more limited gathering takes place to capture missed or new issues as well as potential problems for the following day.

LEVEL 3: LEVEL LOADING, JUST-IN-TIME, BUILT-IN QUALITY

One construct of the pillars emphasizes level loading the work, just-in-time production, and built-in quality. The middle pillar, level loading the work, contains a number

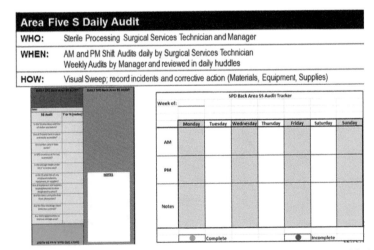

Fig. 10. Tool to support the "sustain" in a 5S project. (*Courtesy of* Oregon Health & Science University, Portland, OR.)

Table 2
The levels and steps of the 5S process

Phase	Level	Sort	Simplify	Sweep	Standardize	Sustain
Continuing operations	Level IV *Improve reliability*	• All areas prone to accumulated clutter identified • Preventive action in place to systematically identify and remedy cause for unneeded items for all areas	• Needed items continuously minimized in number • All needed items can be retrieved within 30 s	• Work area inspection occurs on every shift • Work area supplies and equipment are restocked and well organized	• All members of work group adhere to reliable methods and standards	Work group: • Routinely discusses source and frequency of problems • Identifies root causes and takes corrective action
5S event	Level III *Make it visual*	• MESS prevention strategies are in place • Source of unneeded items tracked	• Needed items outlined • Dedicated locations labeled • Required quantities documented	• Work group agrees on items to be checked • Housekeeping responsibilities and schedule assigned and posted	• All work area procedures are documented and reliably updated	Work group: • Conducts daily audits • Assigns issues to work • Uses 5S board to track issues
	Level II *Focus on the basics*	• Needed and unneeded items are identified • Unneeded items are moved out of the 5S area	• Needed items are stored and organized according to frequency of use	• Visual controls and indicators established to differentiate normal from abnormal work area conditions at a glance	• Work group begins documenting agreements for standard work area procedures	• Audit results posted on communication board in work area • 5S included in orientation and ongoing staff training
As-is operations	Level I *Document a baseline*	• Necessary and unnecessary items intermingled throughout work area	• Needed items located throughout work area	• Key work items missing • Difficult to differentiate normal from abnormal work area conditions	Any work area procedures are: • Undocumented • Inconsistently followed	• No regular work area checks • No measurement of 5S performance

Courtesy of Joan Wellman & Associates, Inc, ©2015; with permission.

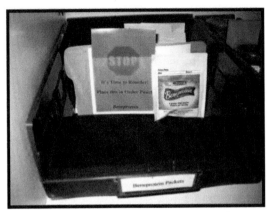

Fig. 11. Ordering signals. Clear trigger to reorder. (*Courtesy of* Oregon Health & Science University, Portland, OR.)

of important concepts. This is scalable. It can relate to hospital census over the course of the year, to the pace of hospital admissions over the course of the day, to antici-pated admissions into the postoperative recovery unit, and to assigning patients to nurses or physicians. The simple principle is that everyone should be fully engaged throughout their shift without being overburdened. Waiting for the next task is an obvious waste. Conversely, being rushed leads to defects (also known as complica-tions). Designing workflows that use everyone optimally can be challenging, but it is also worth pursuing.

One approach to level loading is to redistribute the workload. For example, if the circulating nurses have too many tasks associated with room turnovers, it may be possible to reassign some of them to the surgical technician or the preoperative nurse.

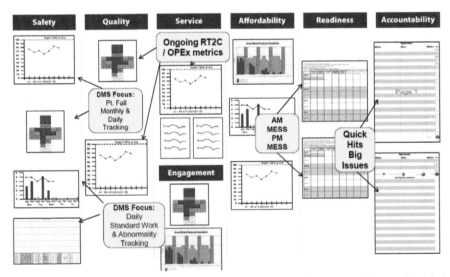

Fig. 12. Visibility board showing the status of lean objectives. (*Courtesy of* Oregon Health & Science University, Portland, OR.)

SOR 0830 Department MESS

	6A	SOR	Scheduling	Anesthesia Support	SPD	Materials	Implants	Departmment Equipment	Epic
Methods									
Comments									
Equipment									
Comments									
Supplies									
Comments									
Staffing									
Comments									

Fig. 13. Daily readiness board for inpatient OR built around methods, equipment, supplies, and staff (MESS). (*Courtesy of* Oregon Health & Science University, Portland, OR.)

Another approach to level loading is to optimize the work itself. In simple terms, one can only achieve level loading if the demand and processes are understood. To accomplish this not so simple task, a number of concepts need to be used. These include the basic lean time concepts of TAKT time and cycle time, standard work, and pull versus push flow.

TAKT time is a measure of the average time required to complete the number of products (or procedures, or visits) demanded by the customer (patient). As a formula it is simply

TAKT Time = Time Available/Number of Procedures

The other important concept is cycle time. This is defined as the time it takes to complete a designated task. When put together, the cycle time needs to be less than the TAKT time or either the tasks will not be completed or the procedures will extend into overtime.

As an example, there are 3 ORs opened for 10 hours each, there are 6 cases that have known times of 1, 3, 3, 5, 6, and 6 hours. The TAKT Time = 10 hours × 3 rooms/6 cases = 5 hours. The cycle time is the 24 hours/6 cases = 4 hours. At a global level, there appears to be enough time to complete all the tasks. There is also apparent opportunity to do more cases on this underutilized day. Even this simple example is subject to complexity. For example, what if the same surgeon has both 6-hour cases? The simple solution may be to adjust block times so that one room is an 8-hour block and another room is a 12-hour block. Another approach would be to focus on these longer cases and see if there is a way to turn them into 5-hour cases.

Patients show up and then often stack up waiting to be seen. Any system trying to optimize the quality of the patient experience will readily admit this is not desirable. Patients, and their conditions, can often be unpredictable. However, most causes of variability between scheduled and actual are from system design or provider behaviors. This includes "optimistically" underestimating cycle times so as to be allowed to schedule the desired number of patients. In academic centers, it is heavily influenced by trainee/learner experience in which early in a rotation the trainee/learner takes longer than at the end of the rotation. Hospitals are filled with additional examples of behaviors and systems that lead to waste. Unpredictable selection of equipment or supplies promotes inefficient activities or workarounds. If a resident is not sure which endotracheal tube is preferred, the resident is likely to prepare several sizes, just in case. The result is wasted time and a wasted tube. Similarly, if it is unclear which instruments a surgeon will request, some combination of waiting for unprepared instruments and having instruments sterilized, delivered, and then returned unused will be the norm.

The lean approach to these problems starts with creating standard work. The process of having standard work allows for measurements to be made. This becomes the basis for improvement. Standard work is often mischaracterized as mindless. In fact, it is exactly the opposite. Standard work is targeted to be the most efficient method to produce a desired result. Identifying that method takes teamwork and analysis.

Physicians tend to emphasize the unique aspects of each patient. This is an important behavior on both a medical and interpersonal level; however, there tends to be more commonalities for most procedures than differences. The more standardization (less variability) there is in a system, the more reliable the system and greater the opportunity to reduce waste. An organization is likely to never fully identify and implement the perfect standard work. Indeed, new medications, procedures, or changes in demand make it a moving target. These are not barriers to implementing standard work because the real question to ask is "will the new standard work better than the current state?"

Initially, standard work reduces average times and it reduces variability. Reducing variability increases predictability and has significant benefits. For example, knowing how long a surgical procedure will take allows for better planning of postoperative staffing, bed assignments, and room turnover resources, as well as predictable times for subsequent patients. For example, increasing the predictability of second case starts can reduce patients' wait times and/or the surgical teams' wait times. Because lean management emphasizes continuous improvement, it is expected to not only maintain the gains made by the standard work but to also identify and implement further gains.

Another lean concept in dealing with patient and material flow is the concept of a pull system. The flow of most steps in health care is push. A patient shows up to the clinic, the blood laboratory, or the radiology area, a box of supplies arrives at a time remote from when it is needed. When flow that uses a push system has a cycle time that exceeds the TAKT time, it causes waiting for patients or inventory accumulation downstream. If it has a cycle time that is much shorter than TAKT time, it causes waiting for the clinicians downstream. Using pull systems instead allows for a much less wasteful process. For inventory, the use of kanban supports processes that minimize unnecessary inventory. The implementation of pull systems is easier to implement for supplies and equipment than it is for patient flow. Once a patient is in the system, he or she needs to be somewhere. Nevertheless, using a pull system allows the patient to wait in the most optimal environment. For example, it is better to be in one's room than on an OR stretcher waiting for surgery.

Just-in-time service is described as providing the right service in the right amount at the right time and right place. In simple terms, it means "no waiting." Working toward just-in-time processes can help emphasize the patient-centric perspective of an organization. Just-in-time is far more than solving the problem of patients waiting for something to happen. It also includes reducing the frequency of surgeons, nurses, or anesthesiologists waiting for each other, equipment arriving too soon and obstructing hallways, or excess supplies waiting to become obsolete. Conversely, it means not waiting for equipment to arrive or supplies to be available. In health care, it is hard to envision just-in-time care. Yet, the benefits are quite clear. It encompasses better management of inventory, including transportation and motion, reduces over-production and overprocessing, and helps focus efforts on producing a defect-free product.

Just-in-time requires many of the same processes as level loading, such as predictable flow from standard work, known cycle, and TAKT times and a reliable pull system. Lack of confidence in a reliable delivery system will result in hoarding. If there is a shortage of any items, hoarding will amplify the problem. When just-in-time is being well used, there is better use of inventory as well as reduction in the other wastes.

One example is the process we used to reduce wasting of syringes. Previously, the expectation was that commonly used syringes (eg, succinylcholine, lidocaine) and emergency resuscitation medications would be obtained by the anesthesia provider during room turnover. Given the effort to have efficient room turnovers, it was a common practice for the provider to obtain a full day's worth of syringes first thing in the morning. This resulted in a large quantity of unused syringes at the end of the day. The distribution system was modified to having these syringes stored and automatically restocked between cases. This ensured that the medications were delivered in time for the next anesthetic and removed the incentive to stockpile at the beginning of the day.

Improving turnover times (rapid changeover) is a common goal of OR management. The associated waste surrounding turnovers is substantial. Fewer cases may be completed in a room reducing efficiency and patient access to care, or the extended time could result in extra expenses. Long turnovers can become strongly reinforcing. For example, a surgeon may become engaged in a different activity during a long turnover and then not be available when needed, causing the rest of the team to then be waiting for the surgeon. Depending on the payer, there may be a distinct difference in the revenue to the hospital where the patient charges commence when the patient enters the room and stop when the patient leaves the room. In a sense during a turnover, the meter is off.

The basic steps to achieving a rapid turnover involve understanding the steps in the process, using 5S to eliminate waste, changing internal procedures (activities that occur during the turnover) to external procedures (activities that occur before or after the turnover), using standard work, optimizing the internal procedures, and then optimizing the external procedures. The process of changing internal to external procedures can produce significant results. It played a significant role in reducing our inpatient turnover times by nearly 20%. One activity that contributed was having better-prepared patients by expanding the use of our preoperative clinic. Fewer patients now need additional tests or workup on the day of surgery. We identify patients who have antibodies and need cross-matched blood so they can arrive early enough to have that step completed before the blood is needed. For rooms using the medical direction model, we have increased our efforts to perform the pre-anesthesia evaluation before the turnover begins. We also used standardized workflow of the team of anesthesia provider, circulating nurse, and surgeon to reduce the frequency of more than one provider trying to spend time with the patient.

Batching is when a process produces outputs in groups. The previous example of collecting all one's medications at the beginning of the day is batching. Similarly, having a fixed OR start time for all of the rooms in an OR suite is an example of batching. Generally, batching is less efficient than a continuous pull system. It is prone to overproduction and accumulation of inventory.

Some batching practices can be more challenging to eliminate than others. For example, it has been suggested that staggering OR starts, when using the medical direction care model, would reduce wait times in the rooms the attending physician did not provide services first. The challenge of staggered starts is threefold. First, there needs to be very reliable first case starts. Even with batch starting, there is typically some variability in the first cases entering a room. We see this even though we have 80% in room on time. On top of the 20% late cases, some cases enter the room early. This makes the existing process look less batchlike. It also underscores the problem of deliberately separating the start times. If the first case is a little behind, it delays the start of the second case. Second, it also makes scheduling providers a challenge. It requires ensuring that the attending anesthesiologist is assigned to rooms that have staggered starts or, conversely, not determining the exact start time for a patient until the assignments are made. Third, there are often other reasons for all of the providers to arrive at the same time, such as conferences, huddles, and other team activities. Thus, delaying some cases with a staggered start strategy, may not actually lead to any overall reduction in waste.

Built-in quality is a lean concept that most transparently relates to medicine. The objective is to get it right the first time and if for any reason that fails to happen, to focus on fixing it immediately. As described previously, the ultimate design for built-in quality is error proofing, a method of making it (nearly) impossible to do it wrong. Furthermore, having "hard stops" on infusion pumps can prevent some errors of over-dosing. Adherence to team pauses plays an important role in preventing errors.

If an error does occur, early identification and intervention are important. Making problems visible when they occur is an important feature of a lean operation. For patients it means that corrective interventions can be initiated sooner. It also provides an opportunity to improve the existing process or implement countermeasures that may reduce the harm of that error. The highly publicized problem of endoscopes causing infections is illustrative of the value of identifying problems. The report allowed a complete revisit of the risk benefit of the scopes as well as an opportunity to make the sterilization process more reliable. One can easily envision the value of having problems like this identified sooner rather than later.

IMPORTANCE OF MANAGEMENT

Lean management does not just happen. Management must be committed to the process. It is difficult to imagine an organization that expects its workers to follow standard work unless management uses leader standard work. In other words, the responsibilities and actions of management need to be as transparent and visible as those of the providers (**Fig. 14**).

It is important to recognize that those in management are as prone to having the same types of concerns about the effectiveness of lean as everyone else in their organization. The same interdependencies of mindset and behavior exist for management.

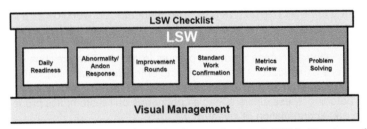

Fig. 14. Sample activities associated with leader standard work (LSW). (*Courtesy of* Oregon Health & Science University, Portland, OR.)

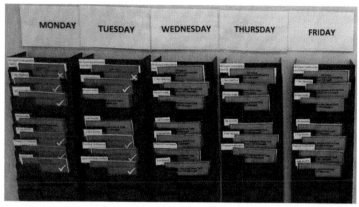

Fig. 15. Example of cards used to display leader standard work. Green represents all metrics were completed, red means some metrics were not met, and blue represents activities pending for later in the week.

To initiate the process of lean management, the leaders must be committed to using lean management tools. If they believe in a system in which every worker is highly valued, they need to back this up by action. From the cultural side, it starts by empowering all employees to feel that they are a part of the solution and their input is taken seriously. Having everyone actively engaged means that management must be actively engaged too.

In lean terms, gemba is where the work is occurring. Therefore, the best way for management to show its visibility is to walk the gemba. Seeing the challenges faced by workers directly has many advantages. One sees problems as they are directly faced by the clinicians and staff, it allows managers to coach and develop important skills, and it allows clinicians and staff a sense that management both cares and "gets it."

The commitment of management is demonstrated when actions are taken to remove barriers to problems, resources are provided to help solve a problem, or time is allocated to clinicians and staff to find solutions. An example of removing barriers can be as simple as authorizing the admitting department to open earlier so patients requiring preoperative regional blocks can be admitted earlier in the morning. Additional resources may be related to providing an analyst to help develop measures of success, which will often include the monetary impact of the changes or trends in satisfaction surveys. Providing time for Kaizen activities requires a major commitment from management. It not only means that employees are given time away from their regular activities, it may mean compensating physicians or advanced providers for their time. More directly, it also requires managers to spend some of their time as active participants in the process.

As with all aspects of lean, visual metrics play a central role in implementation. A leader board readily shows both the findings of the leaders as well as visible evidence of their presence and engagement (**Fig. 15**).

SUMMARY

The basic objectives of medical organizations are truly compatible with the concepts of lean management. Who can argue with a system that is built around safety, quality, service, and affordability? Choosing to use lean management is a significant decision.

It requires a long-term vision and commitment from the organization. When undertaken with commitment and persistence, it can build a culture in which there is engagement and continuous improvement.

REFERENCES

1. Kim CS, Spahlinger DA, Kin JM, et al. Lean health care: what can hospitals learn from a world-class automaker? J Hosp Med 2006;1(3):191–9.
2. Nelson-Peterson DL, Leppa CJ. Creating an environment for care using lean principles of the Virginia Mason Production System. J Nurs Adm 2007;37(6):287–94.
3. Rother M. Toyota Kata: managing people for improvement, adaptiveness and superior results. New York: McGraw-Hill; 2009. p. 297.
4. Liker J. The Toyota way: 14 management principles from the world's greatest manufacturer. New York: McGraw-Hill; 2004. p. 319.
5. Mann D. Creating a lean culture—tools to sustain lean conversions. Standard work for leaders. 2nd edition. Boca Raton (FL): CRC Press; 2010. p. 271.
6. Albanese CT, Aaby DR, Platchek TS. Advanced lean in healthcare. North Charleston (SC): Library of Congress; 2014. p. 230. ISBN: 1-4961-4189-X.
7. Graban M. Lean hospitals—improving quality, patient safety and employee satisfaction. Boca Raton (FL): CRC Press; 2009. p. 252.
8. Wellman J, Jeffries H, Hagan P. Leading the lean healthcare journey: driving culture change to increase value. New York: Productivity Press; 2010. p. 292.
9. Richardson WC, Berwick DM, Bisgard CJ, et al. Crossing the quality chasm—a new health system for the 21st century. Washington, DC: National Academy Press; 2002. p. 337.
10. ANSI/AAMI/ISO 80369-1. Small bore connectors for liquids and gases in healthcare applications. Part 1: General Requirements. Association for the Advancement of Medical Instrumentation. 4301 North Fairfax Drive, Suite 301, Arlington (VA) 22203-1633. 2010. Available at: www.aami.org.
11. Venkataraman-Rao P. US Department of Health & Human Services, Food and Drug Administration, Center for Devices and Radiological Health, Office of Device Evaluation Division of Reproductive, Gastro-renal, and Urological Devices, Gastroenterology Devices Branch. Safety considerations to mitigate the risks of misconnections with small-bore connectors intended for enteral applications. Guidance for Industry and Food and Drug Administration Staff. 2015.

Providing Value in Ambulatory Anesthesia in 2015

Caroline D. Fosnot, DO, MS[a],*, Lee A. Fleisher, MD, FACC, FAHA[b],
John Keogh, MD[c]

KEYWORDS

- Ambulatory anesthesia • Regional anesthesia • PONV • PDNV • OSA • DM

KEY POINTS

- Ambulatory anesthesia's popularity continues to increase and anesthetic techniques will continue to morph and adapt to the needs of patients seeking ambulatory surgery.
- Alterations in already existing medications are promising because these modifications allow for quicker recovery from anesthesia or minimization of it's already known undesirable side effects.
- Postoperative nausea and vomiting, pain, obstructive sleep apnea, and chronic comorbidities are perioperative concerns in ambulatory settings.
- Regional anesthesia has multiple advantages over general anesthesia, providing a minimal recovery period and a decrease in postanesthesia care unit stay.
- Implementation of the Affordable Health Care Act affects ambulatory settings specifically as the demand and need for patients to have screening procedures with anesthesia increases.

Ambulatory anesthesia continues to be in high demand for many reasons: it provides value to patients and surgeons because both parties want their procedure to be swift, involve minimal postoperative pain, have a transient recovery time, and avoid an admission to the hospital. Factors that have made this possible for patients are improved surgical equipment, volatile anesthetic improvement, ultrasound-guided regional techniques, nonnarcotic adjuncts for pain control, and the minimization of postoperative nausea and vomiting (PONV). The decrease in time spent in a hospital also decreases the risk of wound infection, minimizes missed days of work, and is a

Conflicts of Interest: There are no conflicts of interest.
[a] Department of Anesthesiology & Critical Care, Hospital of University Pennsylvania, Perelman School of Medicine, University of Pennsylvania School of Medicine, University of Pennsylvania, 3400 Spruce Street, Dulles Building, 7th Floor, Suite 700, Philadelphia, PA 19104, USA; [b] Perelman School of Medicine of the University of Pennsylvania, Philadelphia, PA 19104, USA; [c] Department of Anesthesiology & Critical Care, Perelman School of Medicine, University of Pennsylvania School of Medicine, Dulles Building Suite 680, Philadelphia, PA 19104, USA
* Corresponding author.
E-mail address: fosnotc@uphs.upenn.edu

Anesthesiology Clin 33 (2015) 731–738
http://dx.doi.org/10.1016/j.anclin.2015.07.011
1932-2275/15/$ – see front matter © 2015 Elsevier Inc. All rights reserved.

socioeconomically favorable model, when possible. Recently proposed strategies that will allow surgeons and anesthesiologists to continue to meet the growing demand for a majority of surgical cases being same day include pharmacotherapies with less undesirable side effects, integration of ultrasound-guided regional techniques, and preoperative evaluations in appropriate candidates via a telephone call the night before surgery. Multidisciplinary communication among caregivers continues to make ambulatory settings efficient, safe, and economically favorable.

It is also important to note the future impact that health care reform will have specifically on ambulatory anesthesia. The enactment of the Patient Protection and Affordable Care Act of 2010 will allow 32 million more people to gain access to preventative services that will require anesthesia, such as screening colonoscopies.[1,2] With this projected increase in the demand for anesthesia services nationwide comes the analysis of its financial feasibility. Some early data looking at endoscopist-administered sedation concludes that It offers greater patient satisfaction, fewer adverse effects than anesthesiologist-administered sedation, and economically advantages. This and future retrospective studies will help to guide health care policy-makers and physicians to come to a conclusion about providing ambulatory services for these millions of patients, but may require confirmation in prospective studies.

The notion that ambulatory anesthesia is an emerging and modern concept is incorrect; since the birth of anesthesia in the 1840s, the first published accounts of successful anesthetics in patients was on an outpatient basis.[3,4] As anesthesia delivery and surgical techniques improved in the mid nineteenth century, both the medical and dental communities used anesthesia for their minor office-based procedures and for tooth extractions, but the use of anesthetics was not deemed appropriate for ill or hospitalized patients quite yet.[4] The marriage of improved operative interventions and anesthetic delivery made for faster recovery and this combination gave way to the 'same-day' or ambulatory surgery concept as we know it today.[5]

Anesthesiology as a medical specialty has matured profoundly since its rudimentary beginning in the mid nineteenth century. Consistent with the advancements in the field of anesthesiology have been the technologic improvements in operative techniques and equipment, decreasing skin-to-skin time, decreasing blood loss, and a need for smaller incisions, which decreases the chance of postoperative wound infection. These factors make the popularity of ambulatory surgery widespread as an attractive and safe option for the more than 35 million patients yearly who undergo same-day operative procedures.[6,7] Luckily, these changes have allowed ambulatory anesthesia to satisfy the increasing economic pressure for cost effectiveness and patients' desires to stay out of the hospital. Multiple factors have made the appeal of same-day surgery a lasting one; adjuvants such as nonsteroidal antiinflammatory drugs, improved ultrasound equipment for regional anesthetics, short-acting narcotics, and the use of induction agents with faster recovery profiles.

POSTOPERATIVE NAUSEA AND VOMITING AND POSTDISCHARGE NAUSEA AND VOMITING

One of the oldest, most common and most challenging complaints about receiving general anesthesia is PONV. Despite advances in antiemetics and multimodal approaches to combat PONV, there is a marked discrepancy between the 2 independent factors; postoperative nausea comprises approximately 20% of complaints and vomiting roughly 4%.[1,2,8–11] It is one of the most common complaints from surgical patients and in a subset of high-risk patients with either a known history of PONV or a coexisting history of motion sickness the incidence can be as high as 80%. PONV is uncomfortable for the patient and can cause unanticipated hospital admission and increase the duration of the postanesthesia care unit (PACU) stay.[1,2,8,9]

Key factors in achieving optimal value in ambulatory surgery are prevention of PONV and postoperative pain. Years of collective data from ambulatory surgical settings has furnished the Society for Ambulatory Anesthesia (SAMBA) with enough data to have recently provided 2013 guidelines for the management of PONV and an updated metaanalysis looking at the use of dexamethasone for prevention of PONV.[1,2,8] Despite advances in pain relief, antiemetics, bronchodilators, and the addition of regional anesthetic techniques pain, PONV and respiratory complications remain common and prevalent challenges. The addition and improvement in postoperative pain control is being reduced with the use of adjuncts such as cyclooxygenase inhibitors and nonsteroidal antiinflammatory drugs and regional blocks.[12,13]

Multimodal therapy for PONV remains the most effective strategy and recent research demonstrating the efficacy of the commonly used antiemetic ramosetron for chemotherapy may make it widely available in the future as a promising anti-PONV drug for the outpatient setting.[14,15] Patient satisfaction is still a powerful driving force in the ambulatory setting and the consistent patient satisfaction with regional blocks makes their use not only requested but highly effective from an economic perspective cost effective, as shown in many trials. Recent work by Abdullah's group showed that a combination of total intravenous anesthetics and multilevel paravertebral blocks for breast mass removal in the outpatient setting demonstrated high patient satisfaction, improved quality of recovery, and expedited discharge from the PACU. Ultrasound-guided regional anesthesia continues to provide excellent postoperative pain control, while minimizing the negative effects of continued narcotic use in the recovery phase.

Another component critical to ambulatory surgery is the condition of postdischarge nausea and vomiting (PDNV), which, according to Apfel and colleagues,[8] is more prevalent than PONV. Practically speaking, this is more concerning because the patient has been discharged from medical observation and no longer has access to intravenous fluids or medication, making dehydration, nausea, an inability to eat, and taking oral pain medication impossible.

This group of researchers recently followed more than 2000 patients for 2 days who received general anesthesia in an ambulatory setting and identified 5 independent predictors of an increased risk of developing PDNV.

Apfel and colleagues[8] concluded that there are specific factors associated with an increased risk of PDNV: female sex, age less than 50 years, history of PONV, opioid administration in recovery, and nausea in the PACU. The results found that PDNV is approximately 10%, 20%, 30%, 50%, 60%, or 80% when 0, 1, 2, 3, 4, or 5 of these factors are present, respectively. This dataset is helpful because it provides a quick tool to the anesthesiologist in the preoperative setting. Ambulatory anesthetics can then be tailored to individuals who present multiple risk factors, which still include avoidance of nitrous oxide, narcotics earlier in the procedure and nonopioid adjuncts, such as regional blocks when appropriate, and nonsteroidal antiinflammatory drugs, ketorolac, or acetaminophen in the PACU.

Most guidelines on preventing PONV indicates much of what is currently practiced in ambulatory settings: the use of 4 to 5 mg IV dexamethasone before incision, and that multimodal therapy including transdermal scopolamine, 4 to 8 mg (not to exceed 16 mg/day) ondansetron and total intravenous anesthetics for a patients with a known history of PONV are each additive in the beneficial effects of minimizing PONV and PDNV.

CAN PATIENTS WITH OBSTRUCTIVE SLEEP APNEA BE OPERATED ON IN AN AMBULATORY CARE SETTING?

The ambulatory setting was once considered an inappropriate setting for patients with a diagnosis of OSA; however, recent data suggest that there is no increased morbidity or mortality when patients with OSA need ambulatory procedures; therefore, the economic and patient satisfaction advantages can be realized.[16] The development of the screening STOP-BANG questionnaire (**Fig. 1**) has helped clinicians to quickly capture patients suffering from OSA, and it allows for preoperative planning appropriate for this type of patient.[17] The current consensus statement endorsed by the SAMBA in 2012 is still considered to be the best approach to successfully caring for the patient with OSA in an ambulatory setting.[18]

Strategies used to optimize the OSA patient in an ambulatory setting include continuous positive airway pressure preoxygenation before induction with 100% oxygen, the use of regional techniques when possible, opioid minimization, and the use of oral or nasal airways to prevent obstruction in the PACU.[19]

Height _____ inches/cm Weight _____ lb/kg Age _____ Male/Female BMI _____

Collar size of shirt: S, M, L, XL, or _____ inches/cm Neck circumference[a] _____ cm

1. *Snoring* Do you snore loudly (louder than talking or loud enough to be heard through closed doors)? Yes No

2. *Tired* Do you often feel tired, fatigued, or sleepy during daytime? Yes No

3. *Observed* Has anyone observed you stop breathing during your sleep? Yes No

4. Blood *pressure* Do you have or are you being treated for high blood *pressure?* Yes No

5. *BMI* BMI more than 35 kg/m^2? Yes No

6. *Age* Age over 50 yr old? Yes No

7. *Neck* circumference Neck circumference greater than 40 cm? Yes No

8. *Gender* Gender male? Yes No

[a] Neck circumference is measured by staff *High risk of OSA:* answering yes to three or more items

Low risk of OSA: answering yes to less than three items

Fig. 1. STOP-BANG questionnaire. (Property of University Health Network. www.stopbang. ca. Permission obtained from University Health Network. *Modified from* Chung F, et al. Anesthesiology 2008;108:812–21, Chung, F et al. Br J Anaesth 2012;108:768–75, Chung F, et al. J Clin Sleep Med 2014;10:951–8.)

Currently, Chan and colleagues[16] are reviewing a large historical cohort of data from patients with OSA who underwent noncardiac surgery in an ambulatory setting; analysis of the data will determine whether any vascular complications could be associated with their OSA status. The authors aim to shed light on vascular complications and prevention of these occurrences in noncardiac surgery for patients with OSA; prior studies looked at respiratory and discharge complications, but not vascular complications. Their work will further aid the clinician facing these patients in ambulatory settings.

Although OSA patients pose more of a challenge in the perioperative setting, data continue to show that same-day settings are safe and appropriate for patients with moderate to severe OSA.[18] The STOP-BANG questionnaire is a quick tool to assess undiagnosed patients and it aids the anesthesiologist in preparing for appropriate postoperative monitoring and care. For patients with severe OSA, a thorough preoperative evaluation and a discussion with the surgery team and nursing staff need to assess appropriateness of an ambulatory setting; whether or not to proceed in an outpatient setting is a multidisciplinary one.[19–22]

OPTIMAL CARE FOR PATIENTS WITH DIABETES MELLITUS TYPES 1 AND 2

Despite the worldwide increase in the incidence of diabetes mellitus, there are no current recommendations for glycemic control in the perioperative ambulatory surgery setting. Recent work by Coan and colleagues[23] reaffirmed the need for standardization of glucose monitoring and treatment of blood glucose fluctuations in ambulatory settings. Further work by DiNardo's group[24] found that glycemic control is not protocolized and the anesthesiologist is responsible for monitoring and treating hypo or hyperglycemia. The last large consensus on glucose control in the diabetic ambulatory population was published in 2010, and it concluded that an "optimal" number for glucose levels in ambulatory patients has yet to be established, because the current body of knowledge is targeted at hospitalized populations with different metabolic requirements. An opportunity exists for research in this domain to establish widespread practices for these patients.

OPERATIVE PROCEDURE DURATION, SCOPE, AND "HEALTHSPAN"

In 1976, the *Journal of the American Medical Association* published an article by Patterson and colleagues[25] describing criteria for use of the newly established "Day Op" room at the North Carolina Memorial Hospital, a teaching affiliate of the University of North Carolina School of Medicine, which stated that, "Each patient is charged a standard fee, providing the surgical time does not exceed 1.5 hours...this plus elimination of the usual one- or two-day hospitalization for inpatients decreases hospital costs by approximately 50%." This statement was prudent when the operative procedure length stayed within these confines. Many operative procedures performed in outpatient settings are routinely in excess of 1.5 hours, which adds to recovery room duration of stay, alters fluid management, and can make pain control more challenging. The need for voiding before discharge can require a catheter.[26]

As the population ages and has a longer lifespan, both the number and severity of medical comorbidities requiring cardiovascular medications such as beta-blockers, calcium channel blockers, angiotensin-converting enzyme inhibitors (ACEI) and angiotensin receptor blockers (ARB) also increase.[27] Maintaining health into old age, also referred to as 'healthspan', requires medications and procedures in a population of aged individuals with varying disease burdens.[28] As Burch and colleagues[29] also note that by the year 2017 there will be more people over the age of 65 than under the age of 5 and by 2050 2 of the 9 billion people predicted to be on Earth will be over the age of 60. These patients will require anesthesia for their numerous procedures, surveillance screenings and minor surgeries which are endorsed and encouraged by the U.S. Health and Human Health Services, preventative task force. This poses a challenge to the anesthesiologist in an ambulatory setting who is faced with a complex medical history and the expectation that the preoperative evaluation for these patients will be as comprehensive and swift as with a patient who presents with a fraction of or no medical issues.[30]

SUMMARY

Anesthesiologists continue to create, innovate, and adapt to a rapidly changing medical community. Ambulatory settings continue to be a pleasing and safe option for the patient and for the health care system as a whole and the anesthesiologist can provide value if we can minimize complications and expand the patient population. Both PONV and PDNV remain common complaints, which are amenable to multimodal therapy. The use of ultrasound-guided regional techniques are excellent nonopioid options for postoperative pain relief while decreasing PONV and carrying minimal to zero side effects. Comorbid conditions and an aging population make preoperative planning essential to successful care of these patients. Mild to moderate OSA patients can be cared for in ambulatory settings safely, with proper evaluation, pretreatment, and meticulous airway forecasting. Diabetic patients and their glycemic control remain as an area in the ambulatory setting that requires further investigation. Currently the guidelines for glucose management are from 2010. It would be beneficial worldwide to establish guidelines for glucose control in this population.

ACKNOWLEDGMENTS

The authors thank the perioperative nursing and perioperative staff at the Perelman Center for Advanced Medicine, Hospital of the University of Pennsylvania for their constant input and feedback about the challenges and successes in this outpatient setting.

REFERENCES

1. Gan TJ, Meyer TA, Apfel CC, et al, Department of Anesthesiology, Duke University Medical Center. Consensus guidelines for managing postoperative nausea and vomiting. Anesth Analg 2003;97:62–71.
2. Gan TJ, Meyer TA, Apfel CC, et al. Society for Ambulatory Anesthesia Guidelines for the management of post operative nausea and vomiting. Anesth Analg 2007; 105:1615–28.
3. Urman RD, Desai SP. History of anesthesia for ambulatory surgery. Curr Opin Anaesthesiol 2012;25:641–7.
4. Pregler JL, Kapur PA. The development of ambulatory anesthesia and future challenges. Anesthesiol Clin North Am 2003;21:207–28.
5. Gangadhar SB, Gopal TM, Sathyabhama, et al. Rapid emergence of day-care anesthesia: a review. Indian J Anaesth 2012;56(4):336–41.
6. Whippey A, Kostandoff G, Paul J, et al. Predictors of unanticipated admission following ambulatory surgery: a retrospective case-control study. Can J Anaesth 2013;60:675–83.
7. Eger EI, White PF, Bogetz MS. Clinical and economic factors important to anesthetic choice for day-case surgery. Pharmacoeconomics 2000;17(3): 245–62.

8. Apfel CC, Philip BK, Cakmakkaya OS, et al. Who is at risk for post- discharge nausea and vomiting after ambulatory surgery? Anesthesiology 2012;117:475–86.
9. Gildasio S, Castro-Alves LJ, Ahmad S, et al. Dexamethasone to prevent postoperative nausea and vomiting: an updated meta-analysis of randomized controlled trials. Anesth Analg 2013;116:158–73.
10. Stierer TL, Wright C, George A, et al. Risk assessment of obstructive sleep apnea in a population of patients undergoing ambulatory surgery. J Clin Sleep Med 2010;6:467–72.
11. Bryson GL, Gomez CP, Jee RM, et al. Unplanned admission after day surgery: a historical cohort study in patients with obstructive sleep apnea. Can J Anaesth 2012;59(9):842–51.
12. Liu SS, Strodbeck WM, Richman JM, et al. A comparison of regional versus general anesthesia for ambulatory anesthesia: a meta-analysis of randomized controlled trials. Anesth Analg 2005;101(6):1634–42.
13. Abdallah FW, Morgan PJ, Cil T, et al. Ultrasound-guided Multilevel Paravertebral Blocks and Total Intravenous Anesthesia Improve the Quality of Recovery after Ambulatory Breast Tumor Resection. Anesthesiology 2014;120:703–13.
14. Banerjee D, Das A, Majumdar S, et al. PONV in Ambulatory surgery: a comparison between Ramosetron and Ondansetron: a prospective, double-blinded, and randomized controlled study. Saudi J Anaesth 2014;8(1):25–9.
15. Shapiro FE, Urman RD. Ambulatory surgery and anesthesia: creating a culture of safety in a cost-effective, quality-conscious Environment. American Society of Anesthesiologist Newsletter 2014;(78):5.
16. Chan MT, Wang CY, Seet E, et al. Postoperative vascular complications in unrecognized Obstructive Sleep apnoea (POSA) study protocol: an observational cohort study in moderate-to-high risk patients undergoing non-cardiac surgery. BMJ Open 2014;4(1):e004097.
17. Joshi GP, Ankichetty SP, Gan TJ, et al. Society for Ambulatory Anesthesia consensus statement on preoperative selection of adult patients with obstructive sleep apnea scheduled for ambulatory surgery. Anesth Analg 2012;115(5):1060–8.
18. Baugh R, Burke B, Fink B, et al. Safety of outpatient surgery for obstructive sleep apnea. Otolaryngol Head Neck Surg 2013;148(5):867–72.
19. American Society of Anesthesiologists. Practice guidelines for the perioperative management of patients with obstructive sleep apnea. Anesthesiology 2014;120:1–19.
20. Chung F, Subramanyam R, Liao P, et al. High STOP-bang score indicates a high probability of obstructive sleep apnoea. Br J Anaesth 2012;108(5):768–75.
21. Chung F, Yegneswaran B, Liao P, et al. STOP questionnaire: a tool to screen patients for obstructive sleep apnea. Anesthesiology 2008;108:812–21.
22. Chung F, Liao P, Yegneswaran B, et al. Postoperative changes in sleep-disordered breathing and sleep architecture in patients with obstructive sleep apnea. Anesthesiology 2014;120:287–311.
23. Coan KE, Schlinkert AB, Beck BR, et al. Perioperative management of patients with diabetes undergoing ambulatory surgery. J Diabetes Sci Technol 2013;7(4):983–9.
24. DiNardo M, Donihi AC, Forte P, et al. Standardized glycemic management and perioperative glycemic outcomes in patients with diabetes mellitus who undergo same-day surgery. Endocr Pract 2011;17(3):404–11.
25. Patterson JF, Bechtoldt AA, Levin KJ. Ambulatory surgery in a university setting. JAMA 1976;235(3):266–8.

26. Koenig T, Neumann C, Ocker T, et al. Estimating the time needed for induction of anesthesia and its importance in balancing anaesthetists and surgeons' waiting times around the start of surgery. Anaesthesia 2011;66: 556–62.
27. Smith I, Jackson I. Beta-blockers, calcium channel blockers, angiotensin converting enzyme inhibitors and angiotensin receptor blockers: should they be stopped or not before ambulatory anesthesia? Curr Opin Anaesthesiol 2010;23(6):687–90.
28. Wolf A, McGoldrick KE. Cardiovascular pharmacotherapeutic considerations in patients undergoing anesthesia. Cardiol Rev 2011;19(1):12–6.
29. Burch JB, Augustine AD, Frieden LA, et al. Advances in geroscience: impact on healthspan and chronic disease. J Gerontol A Biol Sci Med Sci 2014;69(Suppl 1): S1–2.
30. Servin FS. Is it time to re-evaluate the routines about stopping/keeping platelet inhibitors in conjunction to ambulatory surgery? Curr Opin Anaesthesiol 2010; 23:691–6.

Acute Pain Management/ Regional Anesthesia

Tiffany Tedore, MD, Roniel Weinberg, MD, Lisa Witkin, MD,
Gregory P. Giambrone, MS, Susan L. Faggiani, RN, BA, CPHQ, Peter M. Fleischut, MD*

KEYWORDS

- Acute pain • Regional anesthesia • Management • Patient satisfaction • Costs

KEY POINTS

- Effective and efficient acute pain management strategies have the potential to improve medical outcomes, enhance patient satisfaction, and reduce costs.
- Pain management track records are having an increasing influence on patient choice of health care providers and will affect future financial reimbursement.
- Dedicated acute pain and regional anesthesia services have been shown to be invaluable components of the efforts to improve acute pain management.
- Nonpharmacologic and alternative therapies, as well as information technology, should be viewed as complimentary to the traditional pharmacologic treatments commonly used in the management of acute pain.
- The use of innovative technologies to improve acute pain management has produced preliminary evidence of efficacy and may be a sound investment for health care institutions.

BACKGROUND

In the United States, 17.9% of gross domestic product is spent on the health care system (approximately $2.7 trillion).[1] Increasing health care costs and an aging population have posed new challenges for health care institutions. In addition, with the introduction of health care reform and a shift in payment structure to pay for performance, further pressure has been placed on the health care system to improve health care quality while reducing costs.

In an attempt to improve patient quality, the Hospital Quality Alliance was formed, which in turn developed the Hospital Consumer Assessment of Healthcare Providers and Systems (HCAHPS) to provide patients with the opportunity to rate the care they receive.[2] These surveys provide a patient perspective regarding 9 key topics: communication with doctors, communication with nurses, responsiveness of hospital staff,

Department of Anesthesiology, Weill Cornell Medical College, 525 East 68th Street, Box 124, New York, NY 10065, USA
* Corresponding author.
E-mail address: pmf9003@med.cornell.edu

Anesthesiology Clin 33 (2015) 739–751
http://dx.doi.org/10.1016/j.anclin.2015.07.005   anesthesiology.theclinics.com
1932-2275/15/$ – see front matter © 2015 Elsevier Inc. All rights reserved.

pain management, communication about medicines, discharge information, cleanliness of the hospital environment, quietness of the hospital environment, and transition of care. With increased attention placed on standardization of patients' perceptions of hospital care, and the adjustment of hospital Medicare payments by the Centers for Medicare and Medicaid Services, health care institutions have become more cognizant of patients' experiences while receiving care and more conscious of the need to ensure patient satisfaction, all at a reasonable cost.

Ineffective postoperative pain management, both acutely and long term,[3–7] has been identified to have an adverse effect on patient satisfaction, as well as on clinical outcomes. Therefore, pain management is the focus of 2 HCAHPS questions. Although satisfaction with pain management has improved over time, this improvement has lagged behind other HCAHPS metrics.[8]

Ineffective postoperative pain management is associated with deep vein thrombosis, pulmonary embolism, coronary ischemia, myocardial infarction, pneumonia, poor wound healing, insomnia,[3] hypertension, tachycardia, and hyperglycemia.[4] Furthermore, high postsurgical pain scores are associated with increased hospital length of stay (LOS), delayed ambulation, long-term functional impairment,[4] the development of chronic postsurgical pain,[6] and physiologic injury.[7] Furthermore, untreated or undertreated acute pain may have implications for long-term effects, including emotional and psychological distress and the transition to pathologic chronic postsurgical pain (CPSP), which is much more difficult to manage. The transition to CPSP is a complex and poorly understood process involving biological, psychological, and social-environmental factors.[9]

Despite the recognition of these adverse events, pain is still a challenge in the postoperative period.[3] A national survey of 250 adults who underwent surgical procedures in the United States revealed that 68% of respondents had moderate, severe, or extreme pain on the day of surgery.[3] Another recent study of 1490 postsurgical inpatients reported moderate to severe postoperative pain in 41% of patients on the day of surgery.[10] In addition, inadequate pain management during a hospital stay has been identified to adversely affect the institution, as well as the patient, through increased readmissions, increased LOS, and poor clinical outcomes. The financial implications related to inadequate pain management have been estimated to affect 100 million adults at a cost of ~$635 billion annually in treatment and lost productivity,[11] causing institutions to refocus their energies on pain management.

With the recent paradigm change in the delivery of surgical care through the perioperative surgical home, the role of anesthesiologists has shifted to have a greater effect on patient care beyond the delivery of anesthetics. Anesthesiologists now have a new role in the coordination of care and the optimization of patient outcomes for the entire surgical continuum.[12] APS teams have expanded beyond postsurgical intervention to include care of inpatients with other types of acute pain, such as that associated with rib fractures, sickle cell crises, and limb ischemia.

A historical perspective on the development of acute pain services and their value is presented in this article. In addition, the value of pain management, regional anesthesia, and alternative therapies is discussed. The article concludes with a discussion of future technologies and the role and value these technologies might play in pain management.

THE VALUE OF AN ORGANIZED ACUTE PAIN/REGIONAL ANESTHESIA SERVICE

Anesthesiologists have been pioneers in the development of APS because of their familiarity with pharmacology, medications, analgesic techniques, regional anesthesia, and involvement with multiple surgical services. Acute pain management is an extension of care already provided by anesthesiologists in operating rooms and the chronic pain outpatient setting.[13] The team approach to postoperative pain management was first proposed ~40 years ago, with a few editorials about these services appearing in the late 1970s.[14] During the late 1980s and early 1990s, a greater focus began to be placed on postoperative pain management with the introduction of guidelines in Australia (1988), the United Kingdom (1990), and the United States (1992).[15,16] Around the same time, Ready and colleagues[17] further developed the concept of the team-based approach into an anesthesiology-based postoperative pain management service. The APS described by Ready and colleagues[17] consisted of an anesthesiologist-led pain service including an anesthesiologist, anesthesia resident/fellow, and a clinical nurse specialist.[17] This group used 2 modalities: intravenous patient-controlled analgesia and epidural opioid analgesia, with an emphasis on postoperative pain management or pain control. Education regarding the APS and the techniques used was essential.[17] The concept of an APS was further expanded by Rawal[18] to help define vital components, including 24-hour coverage by designated personnel, documentation of regular and appropriate assessments, and the encouragement of active participation with surgeons and nurses to develop postoperative protocols and pathways with defined goals for rehabilitation and mobilization. Other components included patient education, teaching programs for nursing, and analysis of various analgesic techniques and their effect on patient satisfaction and cost-effectiveness.

The nurse-based, anesthesiologist-supervised APS serves as another model of an APS. In this system, the anesthesiologist selects the appropriate analgesic technique, usually based on a clinical protocol or pathway. A specialist acute pain nurse (APN) conducts rounds, and an anesthesiologist is immediately available for consultation. The APN helps support and initiate analgesic plans and coordinates implementation with other unit nurses. This model relies heavily on nursing involvement and the ability to modulate care within a prescribed framework.[19] In addition, APS has become more comprehensive to include pharmacists and physical therapists as well.

Since the inception of APS, the prevalence in the acute care setting has expanded dramatically.[20–22] A 2004 survey of Canadian academic centers found that the prevalence of APS increased from 53% in 1993 to 92% in 2004.[20] Similarly, a survey of US hospitals revealed that 74% of responders had an organized APS, with larger hospitals and academic/university hospitals more likely to have an APS.[22] Although the prevalence of APS has increased, surveys have revealed inconsistent definitions of treatment teams, responsibilities, staffing, and training, and thereby the effectiveness of an APS.[21] Further standardization is necessary using evidence-based protocols.

To show the value of an APS, patient satisfaction and cost-effectiveness must be reviewed. When comparing an APS with traditional pain management strategies, it has been shown that an APS is associated with a significant change to patients' postoperative pain ratings and an increase in satisfaction scores.[14] In one study, Stadler and colleagues[23] reviewed the cost-effectiveness of a nurse-based APS and showed a significant reduction in pain and reduction in postoperative complications in specific surgical specialties. The cost of the service was 19 Euros per day, resulting in a cost saving of 351 Euros per postoperative pain day averted (a measure of analgesic efficacy reflecting pain as an indicator for quality of life).[23] Lee and colleagues[24] conducted a randomized, clinical controlled trial comparing the cost and effect of an APS versus conventional analgesic management after major elective surgery. There was no difference in quality of recovery, a 9-item score measuring postsurgical quality of life, pain intensity, and pain on movement on postoperative day 1. However, there was less pain at rest, less interference of pain with daily activities, and a higher global measure of treatment effectiveness in the APS group on postoperative day 1. The cost in the APS group had a mean increase of $46 dollars/patient; however, in the long term, the incremental cost-effectiveness was of greater benefit (savings per patient, $151; confidence interval [95% CI], $87–$546).

There is a paucity of literature regarding the services that an APS should provide and their cost-effectiveness.[13] In addition, the model of APS that is most effective and will provide the greatest cost benefit is not well established.[25] A review by Lee and colleagues[25] concluded that there was insufficient evidence to conclude whether an anesthesiologist-based or nursing-based APS was more cost-effective. Anesthesia-based/nursing support APS costs ranged from $31.73 to $100.37/patient/d, whereas nurse-based/anesthesiologist-supervised APS ranged from $3.70 to $50.77/patient/d. Cost savings were reflected in shorter intensive care unit stays of $9.90/patient/d, decreased hospital LOS of $11.40/patient/d, and reduction in ward nursing care.[25]

The decision related to which APS model provides the greatest value may depend on the location and size of the hospital.[13] In general, evidence suggests that the establishment of an APS can improve patient satisfaction related to pain and provide cost savings.[14,23,24] Nevertheless, regardless of the specific construct, an APS requires active surgeon cooperation to ensure success.[26] In addition, providing pain medicine training to ward nurses can help facilitate more effective patient care. Ferrell and colleagues[27] described the development and implementation of a pain resource nurse (PRN) program, a 40-hour nursing education program for selected ward nurses to improve pain management in their patient care areas.[28] The nurses in a PRN program are trained in pain assessment and management, and are expected to provide leadership in pain management to other staff on the unit. The objective of the program is to have the PRN nurses model effective pain management, become patient advocates, serve as a resource for clinical decisions, implement pain management projects, and help facilitate patient care with other health care providers, such as the APS.[27,28]

Value of Regional Anesthesia to Patients

There is a large body of literature showing that regional anesthesia and analgesia, both neuraxial and peripheral blockade, decrease pain, as well as postoperative nausea and vomiting.[29–32] For ambulatory surgical patients, regional anesthesia has been proved to result in significantly faster discharge and reduced hospital costs compared with general anesthesia because of the increased ability of patients to bypass the postanesthesia care unit (PACU), shorter PACU stays, and decreased nursing costs.[33,34] Williams and colleagues[33] showed that PACU bypass after anterior cruciate ligament reconstruction resulted in a cost saving of 12%, or $420 per patient. Furthermore, ambulatory continuous peripheral nerve block infusions have been identified to extend the duration of analgesia and result in high patient satisfaction.[35–37]

Regional analgesia with continuous peripheral nerve catheters has shown a similar benefit in inpatients receiving total joint replacement. In a study of patients having total shoulder arthroplasty, Ilfeld and colleagues[38] showed that patients receiving a continuous interscalene infusion met discharge criteria in a median (10th and 90th percentiles) of 21 hours (16–41 hours) compared with 51 hours (37–90 hours) in the control group. Some centers are sending select patients home with continuous peripheral infusions after total joint arthroplasty. Ilfeld and colleagues[39] showed a 14% cost reduction (from $39,100 to $33,646) with ambulatory continuous femoral nerve block infusions in patients after total knee arthroplasty. The patients or their caregivers can typically manage ambulatory nerve block infusions with only a daily phone call from a health care provider. Patients sent home with these infusions report a high rate of satisfaction.[35–37]

Morbidity, Mortality, and Outcome Benefits

Surrogate end points, such as pain scores, opioid consumption, prevalence of post-operative nausea and vomiting, and measures of patient satisfaction, have also been examined. Although these end points are important, they tell clinicians little of the value contributed by regional anesthesia/analgesia to reductions in morbidity and mortality, or to improvements in quality of life. Well-conducted studies examining the impact of regional anesthesia on morbidity and mortality are sparse. Many of the meta-analyses and Cochrane Reviews are based on smaller studies of questionable methodology, and overall show an equivocal effect of regional anesthesia/analgesia on mortality. However, regional anesthesia/analgesia is superior for pain control and may have some benefits for the prevention of respiratory complications and delirium.[40–46]

Some recent, well-conducted database studies examining information from large numbers of patients show multiple benefits from the use of regional anesthesia in patients having orthopedic surgery. Neuman and colleagues[47] showed that regional anesthesia was associated with lower adjusted odds of mortality (odds ratio [OR], 0.710; 95% CI, 0.541, 0.932) and fewer pulmonary complications (OR, 0.752; 95% CI, 0.637, 0.887) compared with general anesthesia in a retrospective cohort of 18,158 patients undergoing hip fracture surgery. A subsequent, retrospective cohort study of 56,729 patients undergoing hip fracture surgery, also by Neuman and colleagues,[48] showed no significant difference in mortality but did show a shorter LOS with regional anesthesia. Memtsoudis and colleagues[49] examined 528,495 patients after total hip and knee arthroplasty and found a 45% reduction in 30-day mortality in those undergoing total knee arthroplasty with regional anesthesia, compared with general anesthesia. In addition, regional anesthesia was associated with significant decreases in morbidity affecting various organ systems in the total joint arthroplasty population. In a separate study, Memtsoudis and colleagues[50] showed significantly fewer complications in patients with obstructive sleep apnea undergoing total hip or knee arthroplasty with regional anesthesia compared with general anesthesia.

There has been increasing interest in the effects of regional anesthesia and analgesia on cancer recurrence and survival. It is well established that surgery induces a stress response, and that this stress response can impair immune system function. Regional anesthesia has been shown to blunt the surgical stress response.[51] There is a large volume of basic science and animal research showing that volatile anesthetic agents and opiates suppress the immune system and/or promote tumor cell migration and proliferation.[51,52] There is also evidence showing that local anesthetics are cytotoxic to cancer cells in vitro.[53] Some retrospective studies have shown a benefit of regional anesthesia and/or analgesia compared with general anesthesia and/or traditional opioid-based analgesia, whereas others have shown an equivocal difference between the two in terms of cancer recurrence and survival.[54–60] It is difficult to draw conclusions from retrospective studies because of confounding and bias. Only well-conducted, large, prospective, randomized controlled trials will answer the question as to whether anesthesia and analgesia have an impact on cancer survival or recurrence.

COMPLIMENTARY TOOLS TO ADD VALUE TO ACUTE PAIN AND REGIONAL ANESTHESIA SERVICES

Health care practitioners depend heavily on opioid therapies to treat pain. Although opioids are very effective, patients may develop side effects, including constipation, urinary retention, nausea, sedation, respiratory depression, myoclonus, delirium, sexual dysfunction, and hyperalgesia.[61] Patients with documented opioid-related adverse events have been found to incur statistically significant higher adjusted mean costs, longer mean LOS, and increased readmission rates.[62] Opioid therapy can be detrimental to patients; alternative/nonpharmacologic therapies have therefore been used to enhance pain management.

The concept of multimodal analgesia remains a cornerstone of modern postoperative pain management. Providing analgesia via a combination of analgesic techniques, targeting different pain receptors and pathways in the peripheral and central nervous systems, can have a synergistic effect on analgesia while reducing side effects and doses.[63] This concept uses the addition of peripheral and neuraxial regional techniques, local anesthetics, nonsteroidal antiinflammatory drugs, alpha-2-adrenergic agonists (clonidine), N-methyl-D-aspartate receptor antagonists (ketamine), acetaminophen, and adjuvants such as antiepileptics, certain antidepressants, and benzodiazepines to opioid-based analgesic techniques.

Enhanced Recovery After Surgery programs have addressed the key factors that delay postoperative recovery and prolong hospital stay, including parenteral opioid analgesia, the need to maintain intravenous fluids because of gut dysfunction, and bed rest secondary to lack of mobility.[64] In addition to multimodal analgesia, including regional and neuraxial anesthesia techniques, nonpharmacologic techniques have gained popularity in recent years, many of which are generally low risk and offer potentially valuable additions to pharmacologic modalities.[64]

Complementary and Alternative Medicine

Complementary and alternative medicine is used as an adjunct therapy with standard pain management techniques and is generally considered to be of low toxicity.[65] These nonpharmacologic therapies may prove beneficial, especially in patients who are difficult to manage, such as children, patients with chronic pain, and patients with multiple medication intolerances. The incorporation of alternative forms of pain management, including education, relaxation techniques, hypnosis, music therapy, transcutaneous electrical nerve stimulation (TENS), guided imagery, biofeedback, and acupuncture, may improve the management of acute pain.[66]

The benefits of nonpharmacologic interventions have shown mixed evidence.[64] A recent study by Bao and colleagues[65] identified no benefits for acupuncture (vs drug therapy or sham acupuncture), and inconsistent results related to massage therapy, TENS, and *Viscum album* L plus cancer treatment. In contrast, acupuncture is gaining acceptance because additional studies are showing potential benefits in both acute and chronic pain and cost-effectiveness compared with routine care.[67–69] A systematic review of the effectiveness of acupuncture after back surgery, as well as orthopedic surgery, identified encouraging but limited evidence.[68] The pain-relieving properties of acupuncture postoperatively in several clinical settings have been shown.[70] Although acupuncture has been used for acute pain management in Japan since the 1970s with good efficacy, detailed examinations still need to be conducted to clarify treatment, dose, timing of treatment, and the propriety of acupuncture treatment.[71]

Music therapy has been identified as having a positive effect on quality of life, with less pain reported posthospitalization compared with control patients.[72] Additional studies have identified the benefits of music therapy in reducing levels of anxiety.[73] Furthermore, Onieva-Zafra and colleagues[74] identified a statistically significant difference in mean pain severity score among patients with fibromyalgia who listened to music for 60 minutes compared with the control group who did not listen to music. In addition, the investigators of a Cochrane Review concluded that listening to music reduces pain intensity and opioid requirements.[75] Overall, it seems that music therapy is an inexpensive, noninvasive technique with no side effects that has an effective role in physical, psychological, social, emotional, and spiritual recovery.[76] Moreover, there is moderate evidence that listening to known and liked music may decrease disease burden and enhance the immune system by modifying stress.[77] The true value of these techniques in preventing/reducing patient pain levels and improving patient outcomes and satisfaction has not been fully realized or described. Therefore, additional research showing efficacy of these nonpharmaceutical interventions is needed.

Information Technology

In addition to nonpharmacologic/alternative treatment of acute pain, information technology provides APS with opportunities to monitor and treat patients in innovative ways. With the proliferation of new technologies and instantaneous data exchange, the global health care system is consistently under pressure to reduce health care costs, maintain high efficiency and quality of care, and remain up to date technologically. Because of health care shortages in the setting of an aging population and improved access to care, external pressure, and regulations from government agencies to reduce costs, the health care system must find a way to improve the quality of patient care with workforce shortages.[78,79] Therefore, in this shifting environment, APS must continue to use/embrace innovative medical technologies and become more efficient in the collection and analysis of this information to improve patient quality and value.

In the realm of pain medicine, much research has been conducted regarding the use of innovative technologies to reduce pain, including the integration of mobile technologies. With the proliferation of the mobile smartphone market (approximately 75% of the mobile phone market as of December 2014),[80] and the potential to collect information on pain status cost-effectively, clinicians have the ability to monitor patients' pain statuses remotely while the patients engage in their daily activities.[81] This information provides great value to treating clinicians, as well as patients, by assisting in clinician decision making; promoting positive, real-time feedback regarding behavioral changes; and enhancing the provider-patient relationship through effective communication.[81]

These data may be collected actively or passively. Active data collection requires input from the patient or user, whereas passive data collection occurs in the background of the smartphone device and transmits these data to an authorized user.[81] Each data collection method has advantages, and may depend on the population served and a patient's ability to actively participate in pain monitoring.[81] In addition, these devices may be used to facilitate the delivery of interventions, such as methods of chronic and acute pain management.[81] The use of mobile technologies and applications to manage chronic conditions has been shown to have value to patients and providers.[82–84] However, few studies have shown the feasibility/effectiveness of smartphone applications for the remote monitoring of patients acutely.

Semple and colleagues[85] used a mobile application to monitor the postoperative pain status of patients at home. During the study period, enrolled subjects were asked to use a mobile phone daily for 30 days to complete a quality-of-recovery scale and take pictures of the surgical site. To assess progress, a surgeon reviewed data daily. This study had 2 key findings. First, Semple and colleagues[85] showed that patient mobile phone monitoring was feasible for patients and effective at detecting complications. Second, provider and patient satisfaction, as well as adherence in this acute postoperative population, were high.

With advancements of mobile technologies and the growing evidence of their benefit in patient management,[82–85] there has been an increased interest in the development of smartphone applications related to pain management. A recent review found 111 mobile applications designed for pain management/education; however, physician involvement in the development of these applications was low.[86] To understand the full value of the use of mobile technologies in pain management, further study is needed. In addition, greater physician involvement in the development of these technologies is essential to ensure that patients are monitored appropriately and receiving the most accurate information to help manage symptoms and promote healthy lifestyle changes.

In addition to the successes of mobile technologies, the use of telemedicine has shown positive results related to pain management.[87–89] Telemedicine allows the provision of health care services to patients who are not in close proximity to a health care facility or provider. However, to provide these services, the appropriate technologies are required (ie, high-speed Internet and high-bandwidth telecommunication systems).[88] The use of telemedicine has shown positive value both financially and in patient satisfaction, with a ~70% reduction of median patient costs and an increase in satisfaction (56% of patients receiving telemedicine were highly satisfied compared with 24% of the in-person patients).[88] The implementation of telemedicine has great potential in acute pain management, including improved access and continuity of care at great distances, medical and surgical follow-up, and preventative medicine and patient education.[89]

A more recent innovation in pain management has been the implementation of virtual reality (VR), allowing patients to engage themselves in this multisensory technology, potentially decreasing perception of pain.[90] However, research regarding VR implementation in pain management is new and although investigations have shown initial promise, additional studies with greater scientific rigor, larger sample sizes, and sound methodology are necessary.[90,91]

SUMMARY

Effective and efficient acute pain management strategies have the potential to improve medical outcomes, enhance patient satisfaction, and reduce costs. Pain management track records are having an increasing influence on patient choice of health care providers and will affect financial reimbursement in the future. Dedicated acute pain and regional anesthesia services have been shown to be invaluable components of the efforts to improve acute pain management. In addition, nonpharmacologic and alternative therapies, as well as information technology, should be viewed as complimentary to the traditional pharmacologic treatments commonly used in the management of acute pain. The use of innovative technologies to improve acute pain management has shown preliminary evidence of efficacy and may be a sound investment for health care institutions.

REFERENCES

1. FastStats - Health expenditures. 2014. Available at: http://www.cdc.gov/nchs/fastats/health-expenditures.htm. Accessed February 17, 2015.
2. Gupta A, Daigle S, Mojica J, et al. Patient perception of pain care in hospitals in the United States. J Pain Res 2009;2:157–64. Available at: http://www.ncbi.nlm.nih.gov/pmc/articles/PMC3004628/. Accessed February 17, 2015.
3. Apfelbaum JL, Chen C, Mehta SS, et al. Postoperative pain experience: results from a national survey suggest postoperative pain continues to be undermanaged. Anesth Analg 2003;97(2):534–40. table of contents. Available at: http://www.ncbi.nlm.nih.gov/pubmed/12873949. Accessed February 10, 2015.

4. Wu CL, Raja SN. Treatment of acute postoperative pain. Lancet 2011;377(9784): 2215–25.
5. Morrison RS, Magaziner J, McLaughlin MA, et al. The impact of post-operative pain on outcomes following hip fracture. Pain 2003;103(3):303–11. Available at: http://www.ncbi.nlm.nih.gov/pubmed/12791436. Accessed February 17, 2015.
6. Macrae WA. Chronic post-surgical pain: 10 years on. Br J Anaesth 2008;101(1): 77–86.
7. Carr DB, Goudas LC. Acute pain. Lancet 1999;353(9169):2051–8.
8. Gupta A, Lee LK, Mojica JJ, et al. Patient perception of pain care in the United States: a 5-year comparative analysis of hospital consumer assessment of health care providers and systems. Pain Physician 2014;17(5):369–77. Available at: http://www.ncbi.nlm.nih.gov/pubmed/25247895. Accessed February 17, 2015.
9. Clarke H, Woodhouse LJ, Kennedy D, et al. Strategies aimed at preventing chronic post-surgical pain: comprehensive perioperative pain management after total joint replacement surgery. Physiother Can 2011;63(3):289–304.
10. Sommer M, de Rijke JM, van Kleef M, et al. The prevalence of postoperative pain in a sample of 1490 surgical inpatients. Eur J Anaesthesiol 2008;25(4):267–74.
11. Institute of Medicine (US) Committee on Advancing Pain Research, Care, and Education. Relieving pain in America: a blueprint for transforming prevention, care, education, and research. Washington, DC: National Academics Press; 2011. Available at: http://www.ncbi.nlm.nih.gov/pubmed/22553896.
12. Cyriac J, Cannesson M, Kain Z. Pain management and the perioperative surgical home: getting the desired outcome right. Reg Anesth Pain Med 2015; 40(1):1–2.
13. Sun E, Dexter F, Macario A. Can an acute pain service be cost-effective? Anesth Analg 2010;111(4):841–4.
14. Werner MU, Søholm L, Rotbøll-Nielsen P, et al. Does an acute pain service improve postoperative outcome? Anesth Analg 2002;95(5):1361–72. table of contents. Available at: http://www.ncbi.nlm.nih.gov/pubmed/12401627. Accessed February 23, 2015.
15. Upp J, Kent M, Tighe PJ. The evolution and practice of acute pain medicine. Pain Med 2013;14(1):124–44.
16. Boezaart AP, Munro AP, Tighe PJ. Acute pain medicine in anesthesiology. F1000Prime Rep 2013;5:54.
17. Ready LB, Oden R, Chadwick HS, et al. Development of an anesthesiology-based postoperative pain management service. Anesthesiology 1988;68(1): 100–6. Available at: http://www.ncbi.nlm.nih.gov/pubmed/3337359. Accessed February 23, 2015.
18. Rawal N. 10 years of acute pain services–achievements and challenges. Reg Anesth Pain Med 1999;24(1):68–73. Available at: http://www.ncbi.nlm.nih.gov/pubmed/9952098. Accessed February 23, 2015.
19. Rawal N. Organization, function, and implementation of acute pain service. Anesthesiol Clin North America 2005;23(1):211–25.
20. Goldstein DH, VanDenKerkhof EG, Blaine WC. Acute pain management services have progressed, albeit insufficiently in Canadian academic hospitals. Can J Anaesth 2004;51(3):231–5.
21. Harmer M. When is a standard, not a standard? When it is a recommendation. Anaesthesia 2001;56(7):611–2. Available at: http://www.ncbi.nlm.nih.gov/pubmed/11437758. Accessed February 23, 2015.
22. Nasir D, Howard JE, Joshi GP, et al. A survey of acute pain service structure and function in United States hospitals. Pain Res Treat 2011;2011:934932.

23. Stadler M, Schlander M, Braeckman M, et al. A cost-utility and cost-effectiveness analysis of an acute pain service. J Clin Anesth 2004;16(3):159–67.
24. Lee A, Chan SKC, Chen PP, et al. The costs and benefits of extending the role of the acute pain service on clinical outcomes after major elective surgery. Anesth Analg 2010;111(4):1042–50.
25. Lee A, Chan S, Chen PP, et al. Economic evaluations of acute pain service programs: a systematic review. Clin J Pain 2007;23(8):726–33.
26. Rawal N. Acute pain services revisited–good from far, far from good? Reg Anesth Pain Med 2002;27(2):117–21. Available at: http://www.ncbi.nlm.nih.gov/pubmed/11915055. Accessed February 23, 2015.
27. Ferrell BR, Grant M, Ritchey KJ, et al. The pain resource nurse training program: a unique approach to pain management. J Pain Symptom Manage 1993;8(8):549–56. Available at: http://www.ncbi.nlm.nih.gov/pubmed/7525784. Accessed February 23, 2015.
28. Ladak SSJ, McPhee C, Muscat M, et al. The journey of the pain resource nurse in improving pain management practices: understanding role implementation. Pain Manag Nurs 2013;14(2):68–73.
29. Hadzic A, Williams BA, Karaca PE, et al. For outpatient rotator cuff surgery, nerve block anesthesia provides superior same-day recovery over general anesthesia. Anesthesiology 2005;102(5):1001–7.
30. Hadzic A, Arliss J, Kerimoglu B, et al. A comparison of infraclavicular nerve block versus general anesthesia for hand and wrist day-case surgeries. Anesthesiology 2004;101(1):127–32. Available at: http://www.ncbi.nlm.nih.gov/pubmed/15220781. Accessed June 5, 2013.
31. Klein SM, Nielsen KC, Greengrass RA, et al. Ambulatory discharge after long-acting peripheral nerve blockade: 2382 blocks with ropivacaine. Anesth Analg 2002;94(1):65–70. table of contents. Available at: http://www.ncbi.nlm.nih.gov/pubmed/11772802. Accessed February 13, 2015.
32. Kettner SC, Willschke H, Marhofer P. Does regional anaesthesia really improve outcome? Br J Anaesth 2011;107(Suppl 1):i90–5.
33. Williams BA, Kentor ML, Vogt MT, et al. Economics of nerve block pain management after anterior cruciate ligament reconstruction: potential hospital cost savings via associated postanesthesia care unit bypass and same-day discharge. Anesthesiology 2004;100(3):697–706. Available at: http://www.ncbi.nlm.nih.gov/pubmed/15108988. Accessed February 13, 2015.
34. Dexter F, Macario A, Manberg PJ, et al. Computer simulation to determine how rapid anesthetic recovery protocols to decrease the time for emergence or increase the phase I postanesthesia care unit bypass rate affect staffing of an ambulatory surgery center. Anesth Analg 1999;88(5):1053–63. Available at: http://www.ncbi.nlm.nih.gov/pubmed/10320168. Accessed February 13, 2015.
35. Ilfeld BM, Enneking FK. Continuous peripheral nerve blocks at home: a review. Anesth Analg 2005;100(6):1822–33.
36. Ilfeld BM, Esener DE, Morey TE, et al. Ambulatory perineural infusion: the patients' perspective. Reg Anesth Pain Med 2003;28(5):418–23. Available at: http://www.ncbi.nlm.nih.gov/pubmed/14556132. Accessed February 13, 2015.
37. Swenson JD, Bay N, Loose E, et al. Outpatient management of continuous peripheral nerve catheters placed using ultrasound guidance: an experience in 620 patients. Anesth Analg 2006;103(6):1436–43.
38. Ilfeld BM, Vandenborne K, Duncan PW, et al. Ambulatory continuous interscalene nerve blocks decrease the time to discharge readiness after total shoulder arthroplasty: a randomized, triple-masked, placebo-controlled study. Anesthesiology

2006;105(5):999–1007. Available at: http://www.ncbi.nlm.nih.gov/pubmed/17065895. Accessed February 13, 2015.

39. Ilfeld BM, Mariano ER, Williams BA, et al. Hospitalization costs of total knee arthroplasty with a continuous femoral nerve block provided only in the hospital versus on an ambulatory basis: a retrospective, case-control, cost-minimization analysis. Reg Anesth Pain Med 2007;32(1):46–54.

40. Parker MJ, Handoll HHG, Griffiths R. Anaesthesia for hip fracture surgery in adults. Cochrane Database Syst Rev 2004;(4):CD000521.

41. Parker MJ, Griffiths R, Appadu BN. Nerve blocks (subcostal, lateral cutaneous, femoral, triple, psoas) for hip fractures. Cochrane Database Syst Rev 2002;(1):CD001159.

42. Guay J, Choi P, Suresh S, et al. Neuraxial blockade for the prevention of postoperative mortality and major morbidity: an overview of Cochrane systematic reviews. Cochrane Database Syst Rev 2014;(1):CD010108.

43. Svircevic V, Passier MM, Nierich AP, et al. Epidural analgesia for cardiac surgery. Cochrane Database Syst Rev 2013;(6):CD006715.

44. Choi PT, Bhandari M, Scott J, et al. Epidural analgesia for pain relief following hip or knee replacement. Cochrane Database Syst Rev 2003;(3):CD003071.

45. Nishimori M, Low JHS, Zheng H, et al. Epidural pain relief versus systemic opioid-based pain relief for abdominal aortic surgery. Cochrane Database Syst Rev 2012;(7):CD005059.

46. Barbosa FT, Jucá MJ, Castro AA, et al. Neuraxial anaesthesia for lower-limb revascularization (Review). Cochrane database of systematic reviews 2013;(7):CD007083.

47. Neuman MD, Silber JH, Elkassabany NM, et al. Comparative effectiveness of regional versus general anesthesia for hip fracture surgery in adults. Anesthesiology 2012;117(1):72–92.

48. Neuman MD, Rosenbaum PR, Ludwig JM, et al. Anesthesia technique, mortality, and length of stay after hip fracture surgery. JAMA 2014;311(24):2508–17.

49. Memtsoudis SG, Sun X, Chiu Y-L, et al. Perioperative comparative effectiveness of anesthetic technique in orthopedic patients. Anesthesiology 2013;118(5):1046–58.

50. Memtsoudis SG, Stundner O, Rasul R, et al. Sleep apnea and total joint arthroplasty under various types of anesthesia: a population-based study of perioperative outcomes. Reg Anesth Pain Med 2013;38(4):274–81.

51. Wolf AR. Effects of regional analgesia on stress responses to pediatric surgery. Paediatr Anaesth 2012;22(1):19–24.

52. Sacerdote P. Opioids and the immune system. Palliat Med 2006;20(Suppl 1):s9–15. Available at: http://www.ncbi.nlm.nih.gov/pubmed/16764216. Accessed February 13, 2015.

53. Chang Y-C, Hsu Y-C, Liu C-L, et al. Local anesthetics induce apoptosis in human thyroid cancer cells through the mitogen-activated protein kinase pathway. PLoS One 2014;9(2):e89563.

54. Exadaktylos AK, Buggy DJ, Moriarty DC, et al. Can anesthetic technique for primary breast cancer surgery affect recurrence or metastasis? Anesthesiology 2006;105(4):660–4. Available at: http://www.pubmedcentral.nih.gov/articlerender.fcgi?artid=1615712&tool=pmcentrez&rendertype=abstract. Accessed February 2, 2015.

55. Biki B, Mascha E, Moriarty DC, et al. Anesthetic technique for radical prostatectomy surgery affects cancer recurrence: a retrospective analysis. Anesthesiology 2008;109(2):180–7.

56. Christopherson R, James KE, Tableman M, et al. Long-term survival after colon cancer surgery: a variation associated with choice of anesthesia. Anesth Analg 2008;107(1):325–32.

57. Gupta A, Björnsson A, Fredriksson M, et al. Reduction in mortality after epidural anaesthesia and analgesia in patients undergoing rectal but not colonic cancer surgery: a retrospective analysis of data from 655 patients in central Sweden. Br J Anaesth 2011;107(2):164–70.

58. Chen W-K, Miao C-H. The effect of anesthetic technique on survival in human cancers: a meta-analysis of retrospective and prospective studies. PLoS One 2013;8(2):e56540.

59. Cummings KC, Patel M, Htoo PT, et al. A comparison of the effects of epidural analgesia versus traditional pain management on outcomes after gastric cancer resection: a population-based study. Reg Anesth Pain Med 2014;39(3):200–7.

60. Cakmakkaya OS, Kolodzie K, Apfel CC, et al. Anaesthetic techniques for risk of malignant tumour recurrence. Cochrane Database Syst Rev 2014;(11):CD008877.

61. Buvanendran A, Kroin JS. Multimodal analgesia for controlling acute postoperative pain. Curr Opin Anaesthesiol 2009;22(5):588–93.

62. Oderda GM, Gan TJ, Johnson BH, et al. Effect of opioid-related adverse events on outcomes in selected surgical patients. J Pain Palliat Care Pharmacother 2013;27(1):62–70.

63. Kehlet H, Dahl JB. The value of "multimodal" or "balanced analgesia" in postoperative pain treatment. Anesth Analg 1993;77(5):1048–56. Available at: http://www.ncbi.nlm.nih.gov/pubmed/8105724. Accessed February 23, 2015.

64. Tan M, Law LS-C, Gan TJ. Optimizing pain management to facilitate Enhanced Recovery After Surgery pathways. Can J Anaesth 2015;62(2):203–18.

65. Bao Y, Kong X, Yang L, et al. Complementary and alternative medicine for cancer pain: an overview of systematic reviews. Evid Based Complement Alternat Med 2014;2014:170396.

66. Rusy LM, Weisman SJ. Complementary therapies for acute pediatric pain management. Pediatr Clin North Am 2000;47(3):589–99. Available at: http://www.ncbi.nlm.nih.gov/pubmed/10835992. Accessed February 12, 2015.

67. Corti L. Nonpharmaceutical approaches to pain management. Top Companion Anim Med 2014;29(1):24–8.

68. Cho Y-H, Kim C-K, Heo K-H, et al. Acupuncture for acute postoperative pain after back surgery: a systematic review and meta-analysis of randomized controlled trials. Pain Pract 2014;15(3):279–91.

69. Lin C-WC, Haas M, Maher CG, et al. Cost-effectiveness of guideline-endorsed treatments for low back pain: a systematic review. Eur Spine J 2011;20(7):1024–38.

70. Chen C-C, Yang C-C, Hu C-C, et al. Acupuncture for pain relief after total knee arthroplasty: a randomized controlled trial. Reg Anesth Pain Med 2015;40(1):31–6.

71. Taguchi R. Acupuncture anesthesia and analgesia for clinical acute pain in Japan. Evid Based Complement Alternat Med 2008;5(2):153–8.

72. Tanabe P, Thomas R, Paice J, et al. The effect of standard care, ibuprofen, and music on pain relief and patient satisfaction in adults with musculoskeletal trauma. J Emerg Nurs 2001;27(2):124–31.

73. Parlar Kilic S, Karadag G, Oyucu S, et al. Effect of music on pain, anxiety, and patient satisfaction in patients who present to the emergency department in Turkey. Jpn J Nurs Sci 2015;12(1):44–53.

74. Onieva-Zafra MD, Castro-Sánchez AM, Matarán-Peñarrocha GA, et al. Effect of music as nursing intervention for people diagnosed with fibromyalgia. Pain Manag Nurs 2013;14(2):e39–46.

75. Bradt J, Dileo C, Grocke D, et al. Music interventions for improving psychological and physical outcomes in cancer patients. Cochrane Database Syst Rev 2011;(8):CD006911.
76. Chlan L, Tracy MF. Music therapy in critical care: indications and guidelines for intervention. Crit Care Nurse 1999;19(3):35–41. Available at: http://www.ncbi.nlm.nih.gov/pubmed/10661090. Accessed February 13, 2015.
77. Pauwels EKJ, Volterrani D, Mariani G, et al. Mozart, music and medicine. Med Princ Pract 2014;23(5):403–12.
78. US Department of Health and Human Services: Health Resource and Services Administration. The registered nurse population. Findings from the 2008 National Sample Survey of Registered Nurses. Rockville (MD): 2010.
79. Projecting the supply and demand for primary care practitioners through 2020. Rockville (MD): US Department of Health and Human Services; 2013. Available at: http://bhpr.hrsa.gov/healthworkforce/supplydemand/usworkforce/primarycare/projectingprimarycare.pdf. Accessed March 4, 2015.
80. Lella A. comScore Reports December 2014 U.S. Smartphone subscriber market share. comScore, Inc; 2015. Available at: http://www.comscore.com/Insights/Market-Rankings/comScore-Reports-December-2014-US-Smartphone-Subscriber-Market-Share. Accessed March 4, 2015.
81. Richardson JE, Reid MC. The promises and pitfalls of leveraging mobile health technology for pain care. Pain Med 2013;14(11):1621–6.
82. Vanderboom CE, Vincent A, Luedtke CA, et al. Feasibility of interactive technology for symptom monitoring in patients with fibromyalgia. Pain Manag Nurs 2014;15(3):557–64.
83. Logan AG, McIsaac WJ, Tisler A, et al. Mobile phone-based remote patient monitoring system for management of hypertension in diabetic patients. Am J Hypertens 2007;20(9):942–8.
84. Irvine AB, Russell H, Manocchia M, et al. Mobile-web app to self-manage low back pain: randomized controlled trial. J Med Internet Res 2015;17(1):e1.
85. Semple JL, Sharpe S, Murnaghan ML, et al. Using a mobile app for monitoring post-operative quality of recovery of patients at home: a feasibility study. JMIR mHealth uHealth 2015;3(1):e18.
86. Rosser BA, Eccleston C. Smartphone applications for pain management. J Telemed Telecare 2011;17(6):308–12.
87. Kroenke K, Krebs EE, Wu J, et al. Telecare collaborative management of chronic pain in primary care: a randomized clinical trial. JAMA 2014;312(3):240–8.
88. Pronovost A, Peng P, Kern R. Telemedicine in the management of chronic pain: a cost analysis study. Can J Anaesth 2009;56(8):590–6.
89. Burton R, Boedeker B. Application of telemedicine in a pain clinic: the changing face of medical practice. Pain Med 2000;1(4):351–7.
90. Mahrer NE, Gold JI. The use of virtual reality for pain control: a review. Curr Pain Headache Rep 2009;13(2):100–9. Available at: http://www.ncbi.nlm.nih.gov/pubmed/19272275.
91. Malloy KM, Milling LS. The effectiveness of virtual reality distraction for pain reduction: a systematic review. Clin Psychol Rev 2010;30(8):1011–8.

Examining Health Care Costs

Opportunities to Provide Value in the Intensive Care Unit

Beverly Chang, MD[a],*, Javier Lorenzo, MD[a],
Alex Macario, MD, MBA[a,b]

KEYWORDS

- US health care costs • Critical care costs • Measuring health care costs
- Fast-track cardiac surgery • Delirium and ABCDE bundle

KEY POINTS

- Increasing health care costs in the United States has mandated a change in current health care spending habits to curb the exorbitant fees needed to provide care for patients.
- Unlike other industries, competition has not aligned cost with value for patients in the health care sector.
- With superior knowledge in postoperative management of sedation, airway, and hemodynamic triaging, anesthesiologists are naturally positioned to be champions for providing value-based care in the postoperative and critical care settings.
- Enacting fast-track cardiac surgery pathways and ABCDE bundles are ways that anesthesiologists can provide optimal value-based care for patients.

THE HEALTH CARE COST CONUNDRUM

The provision and availability of quality health care in the United States have been considered by most to be essential aspects of American life. In recent years, however, the words "health care" have drummed up controversial murmurings of "Obamacare," "the Affordable Care Act," and "health insurance mandates." Since when and why did this basic human need become such a hotly disputed topic?

Currently, more than $2.9 trillion are spent annually on health care, equivalent to $9255 per person per year.[1] National health expenditure projections estimate that

The authors have no disclosures and financial conflicts of interest.
[a] Department of Anesthesiology, Perioperative and Pain Medicine, Stanford University School of Medicine, 300 Pasteur Drive, H3580, Stanford, CA 94305-5640, USA; [b] Department of Health Research and Policy, Stanford University School of Medicine, 300 Pasteur Drive, H3580, Stanford, CA 94305-5640, USA
* Corresponding author.
E-mail address: Bevchang02@gmail.com

Anesthesiology Clin 33 (2015) 753–770
http://dx.doi.org/10.1016/j.anclin.2015.07.012 **anesthesiology.theclinics.com**

health care spending will grow by 5.7% each year until 2022. This outpaces gross domestic product (GDP) growth by 1.1%. By 2023, US national health care spending is expected to reach $4.6 trillion or 19.3% of GDP. In the imminent future, $1 of every $5 in the United States will be spent on health care.[2]

Worldwide, the US health care industry spending equaled the combined spending of the next 10 biggest spenders: China, the United Kingdom, Canada, Germany, France, Japan, Brazil, Australia, Italy, and Spain.[3] This increased spending has little if any added measurable benefit to American healthcare provision and quality when compared with other countries. Higher spending in the United States is not a result of a sicker patient population than compared to other countries; 60% of these expenditures are composed of nondiscretionary costs, which include hospital care (25%), physician and clinical services (26%), and prescription drugs (8%).[4] The remaining 40% consists of the costs associated with long-term care facilities, retail, supervisory care, and administration costs. The United States spends 6 times as much per capita on administration than other countries.[5]

With growing health care expenditures expected from the surge in baby boomers, there is an unprecedented urgency to curb spending. Unless spending is reversed, the federal debt will increase to more than $7.2 trillion by 2022, which equals 70% to 90% of GDP.[6] Health care costs are poised to consume resources at the expense of less funding for schools, parks, roads, and other public needs.

ECONOMICS OF CRITICAL CARE SERVICES

Today, critical care medicine costs up to $80 billion a year, accounting for 3% of all health care costs at nearly 1% of GDP. Intensive Care Unit (ICU) stays cost 3 times the amount of general hospital stays, and up to 26.9% of all hospitalizations include an ICU stay.[7,8] For a majority of medical conditions requiring ICU admissions, ICU charges range from 25% to 38.2% of each patient's aggregate hospital charges (**Box 1**).

The United States devotes more of its hospital resources to critical care medicine than any other country, having the highest ICU bed-to-population and ICU-to–hospital bed ratios in the world.[9,10] More critical care services are provided for elderly and end-of-life care than anywhere else in the world. This demand is expected to increase with the influx of patients entering into the Medicare/Medicaid market and health care exchanges. Currently, Medicare patients who die during admission or within 3 months of discharge were in the upper 25% percentile of ICU resource use; however, higher costs has not been found to be a marker for survival.[11,12]

The bulk of hospital and ICU expenses is overhead costs, otherwise known as fixed expenses, with nursing care constituting the highest portion. The largest fraction of

---

Box 1
ICU statistics in the United States

- 5000 acute care hospitals
- 6500 ICUs with 94,000 beds
- 4 to 8 million patients admitted annually
- Average ICU occupancy rates are 65% to 72% with higher occupancy rates in larger hospitals
- ICU beds account for 15% of hospital beds and represent 13% of hospital expenditures.

Data from Fast Facts on U.S. Hospitals 2015. American Hospital Association; and Utilization of Intensive Care Services, 2011. Healthcare Cost and Utilization Project.

total ICU costs is attributed to the first day of ICU admission and decreases thereafter as acuity decreases. Mechanical ventilation may be the greatest independent predictor of total ICU cost. ICU costs are greater for male patients, surgical patients and trauma patients.[13]

Significant economic and societal costs continue to build even after discharge. Patients' quality of life suffers from loss of strength, nutritional deficits, and cognitive dysfunction once they are discharged after an ICU admission. The losses of productivity as well as cognitive and emotional abilities are important clinical problems that increase long-term downstream costs.

VALUE-BASED HEALTH CARE

In the private sector, competition is the driving force for improvements in the quality and cost of products and services.[14] Companies that produce the best results at the lowest cost are rewarded whereas those that produce inferior products exit the marketplace. This competition however, does not exist in health care despite being the biggest industry in the United States. There is a misalignment between the nature of competition and value for patients in the health care sector.[14] To transform the health care system, including the care of the critically ill, competition and cost need to be realigned with value for patients.[14] The results that all patients truly care about are the outcomes of their medical condition. This is where value should be focused on.[14]

Currently, more than 50% of health care in the United States may be inappropriate, with little or no value added for patients—that is $1.2 trillion of the $2.2 trillion spent on health care in 2008.[15] An estimated 20% to 30% of current health care spending can be saved while providing safe and equal care nationwide (**Figs. 1** and **2**).[16]

Despite the high cost of health care, Americans currently receive only 55% of 30 types of preventive care suggested by current medical standards.[17] Higher cost does not equate to having improved access, better outcomes, higher satisfaction, or reduced mortality.[16] The best care in the United States is unsurpassed but average care is often subpar.[14]

MEASURING HEALTH CARE COSTS

Much of the difficulty in creating a perfect marketplace in the health care industry has been the lack of transparency in health care costs. Unlike for most other industries, the

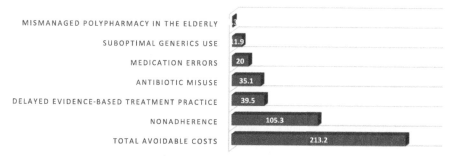

Fig. 1. Estimated avoidable costs in billions of dollars. (*Data from* Avoidable Costs in U.S. Healthcare. The $200 Billion Opportunity from Using Medicines More Responsibly. IMS Institute for Healthcare Informatics. 2013. Available at: http://www.imshealth.com/deployed files/imshealth/Global/Content/Corporate/IMS%20Institute/RUOM-2013/IHII_Responsible_Use_Medicines_2013.pdf. Accessed July 16, 2015.)

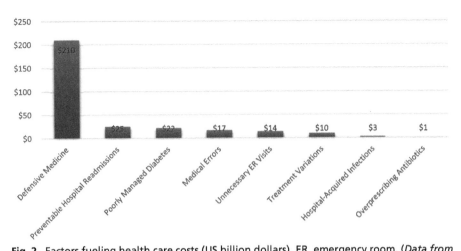

Fig. 2. Factors fueling health care costs (US billion dollars). ER, emergency room. (*Data from* The Price of Excess. Identifying waste in healthcare Spending. PricewaterhouseCoopers Health Research Institute 2010. Available at: http://www.lifesaverapp.com/PDF/PDFsample5.pdf. Accessed July 16, 2015.)

true cost attributed to delivering health care is often unknown. Although charges are known, charge data rarely reflect the true cost to the hospital of providing care. Prices as billed to insurance companies for services do not reflect actual costs. Although direct costs can be estimated from supply costs, cost accounting in hospitals and ICUs needs to be refined to more clearly elucidate the actual costs of health care services.

Charges are often billed from hospital charge masters. These charge masters are every hospital's internal price list, which assigns prices to every service and test provided at the institution. Each billable item must be reflected on the charge master for the hospital to charge for a service or item. The way that each institution arrives at these price assignments however, is neither transparent nor based on true pricing of health care commodities. Cost and charges are not related linearly but are often used interchangeably and thereby incorrectly.[18] Hospital charges are often set over years and updates occur infrequently. Hospitals themselves are often unable to account for the rationale for some of their charges, especially once inflationary increases are applied.[19]

As health care become an increasingly targeted area for cost reduction, the concepts of fixed and variable costs are important terms to understand (**Box 2**).

Box 2
Definitions of fixed and variable costs

- Fixed costs
  - Do not change in proportion to the volume of ICU patients
  - Are incurred regardless of clinical activity
  - Include building/area space costs, equipment, salaried ICU nursing care and salaried pharmacists

- Variable costs
  - Change in relation to number of patients in the ICU
  - Examples include medications, radiographic studies, and laboratory tests
  - Changes in physician prescribing practices in the ICU only affect variable costs

Any cost reduction strategy must take fixed costs into consideration. Decreasing length of stay in the ICU may not necessarily decrease costs if fixed costs are not adequately managed. As patient census in the ICU decreases, average cost per patient increases because fixed costs need to be distributed among fewer patients. When looking at cost reduction strategies, improved care leads to decreased length of stays in the ICU, leading to increased room for new admissions. In fee-for-service reimbursement models, hospital administrators strive to keep hospital and ICUs full to offset fixed costs.

Total medical expenditures can be defined mathematically as the quantity of services delivered (Q) multiplied by the quantity of resources used to produce each service (resources/Q) multiplied by price of the resources (P).

As a result of this formula, it becomes clear that total medical expenditures can only be reduced by 1 or more of 3 mechanisms:

1. Decreasing the amount of medical services delivered. An example is reducing the number of ICU admissions via better public health interventions.
2. Reducing the resources required to deliver a particular patient's care. This (resources/Q) is the inverse of productivity and could be achieved by using resources more efficiently.
3. Reducing the price of the resources (eg, lowering the wages of providers or using a less costly ventilator system to support patients).

Excessive utilization of health care services may be the most important contributor to accelerating costs. To decrease these medical costs, incentives are needed to eliminate unnecessary care. Many medical interventions fall into a gray area in which professional disagreement exists on appropriateness, intensity, and frequency of use. This situation generates some of the practice variation observed.

More selective use of ICU interventions while utilizing those with the highest benefit for cost may result in overall savings. As the pioneers of patient safety, anesthesiologists are positioned to lead these endeavors. With the familiarity of anesthesiologists with airway, ventilator management, pain management, and resuscitation, anesthesiologists are natural providers in the critical care environment.

The remainder of this review focuses on 2 areas in which anesthesiologists can provide value-based care in the ICU: cardiac surgery and delirium management.

CARDIOVASCULAR DISEASE AND CARDIAC SURGERY IN THE UNITED STATES

Heart disease is the leading cause of death in the United States and affects 1 out of every 3 Americans.[20] The total cost (including direct and indirect costs and lost productivity) of managing cardiovascular (CV) disease and stroke in the United States is estimated at $475.3 billion. In comparison, the cost of all cancer and neoplasm treatment in 2010 was $263.8 billion (**Figs. 3** and **4**).[21]

Of the 51.4 million inpatient surgical procedures performed annually, 7.4 million of these procedures are CV procedures.[22] This number increased by 30% between 1996 and 2006. In 2011, coronary artery bypass grafts (CABGs) were the 15th most frequently performed surgical procedure in the nation; 214,000 CABGs were performed that year whereas heart valve procedures were the 20th most frequent, at 120,000.[23] Although recent medical advances have introduced noninvasive medical therapy and procedures to treat cardiac disease, cardiac surgery remains an alternative for patients refractory to medical treatment.

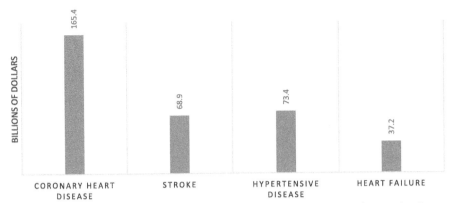

Fig. 3. Estimated direct and indirect costs (US billion dollars) of major cardiovascular disease and stroke, 2009. (*Data from* National Institutes of Health, National Heart, Lung, and Blood Institute. Fact book fiscal year 2009.)

THE COST OF CARDIAC SURGERY

CABG and heart valve procedures were ranked the seventh and eighth most costly procedures performed in 2011, at aggregate costs of $6,411,000,000 and $6,070,000 respectively. Mean cost per hospital stay was $38,700 for CABG and $53,400 for heart valve procedures whereas mean charges were $99,743 and $141,120, respectively.[23] In 2012, the average cost of major cardiac procedures at the Cleveland Clinic was $107,842.[24] In 2015, Steven Brill's follow-up article to the *Time* magazine "Bitter Pill" feature was titled, "What I Learned from my $190,000 Open-Heart Surgery" (**Box 3**).[3,25]

The largest share of costs in this population consisted of operating room personnel staffing (nurses, perfusionists, and physicians) and supplies. ICU costs ranked second below operating room costs.[26–30] A 3-fold cost variation between hospitals suggests

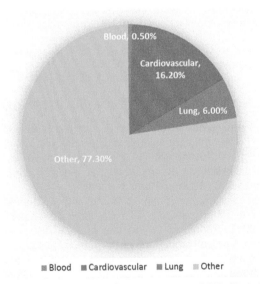

Fig. 4. Percentage of total economic costs by organ system, 2010. (*Data from* National Institutes of Health, National Heart, Lung, and Blood Institute. Fact book fiscal year 2009.)

> **Box 3**
> **Predictors of cost for cardiac surgical patients**
>
> - Increasing patient age
> - ICU and hospital length of stay
> - Intraoperative complications
> - Cardiopulmonary bypass duration
> - Postoperative complications

that standardizing clinical practice across hospitals could incur significant cost savings by increasing efficiency (**Boxes 4** and **5**).[31]

In the postoperative period, duration of mechanical ventilation significantly affects ICU length of stay. Average ICU length of stay is 1.9 days and hospitalization length of stay ranges from 7.1 to 11.6 days. Postoperative events are the greatest determinant of costs and preoperative factors the greatest determinant of hospital length of stay (**Box 6**).[32]

WHAT IS FAST-TRACK CARDIAC SURGERY?

The development of high-dose opioid anesthetics and long-acting paralytics provided a hemodynamically stable anesthetic that transformed the landscape of intraoperative and postoperative cardiac surgical care. Postoperatively however, this translated to prolonged ventilatory support and prolonged ICU stay. These were considered reasonable compromises.

Safer surgical techniques coupled with an increasing elderly population led to an explosive growth in cardiac surgery that outpaced the supply of ICU beds, creating a bottleneck that limited the performance of further surgeries and revenues for hospitals.[33] Fast track for cardiac surgery patients become popular in the 1990s and gained traction rapidly. The idea was to allow for early extubation, thus decreasing ICU stay.

Although there is no standard definition, fast-track cardiac surgery refers to the idea of providing cardiac anesthesia with the goal of extubation within 1 to 6 hours.[34] The implementation of such pathways allows for earlier extubation, shorter ICU stays, decreased hospitalization time, and decreased costs. Although this idea may seem intuitive, historical practices differed vastly, which is why this was viewed as a novel idea when it was introduced.

> **Box 4**
> **Preoperative factors predictive of increased ICU stay and costs**
>
> - Use of intra-aortic balloon pump
> - Congestive heart failure
> - Myocardial infarction
> - Renal failure
> - Obesity
>
> *Data from* Mangano DT. Perioperative cardiac morbidity. Anesthesiology 1990;72:153–84; and Lahey SJ, Borlase BC, Lavin PT. Preoperative risk factors that predict hospital length of stay in coronary artery bypass patients >60 years old. Circulation 1992;86:181–5.

Box 5
Postoperative factors predictive of increased ICU stay and costs after coronary artery bypass graft surgery

- Female
- Nonwhites
- Surgical urgency
- More severe coronary disease
- Duration of mechanical ventilation

Data from Cowper PA, DeLong ER, Peterson ED, et al. Variability in cost of coronary bypass surgery in New York State: potential for cost savings. Am Heart J 2002;143:130–9.

Although there is no standard approach to fast tracking cardiac patients, many institutions have developed specialized protocols that begin in the operating room with the abandonment of traditional cardiac anesthetic techniques. Short-acting hypnotics and opioid medications are used in reduced doses. Postoperatively, patients are brought to the ICU where fast-track ventilator weaning protocols are initiated (**Fig. 5**).

Since the first investigation into fast-track cardiac surgery pathways in the late 1980s, numerous studies have demonstrated their safety and efficacy (**Box 7**).[35,36] A systematic review examining the safety and effectiveness of fast-track cardiac anesthesia demonstrated no evidence of increased mortality or major morbidity rates. Pooled analysis showed a reduction in ICU stay and a shorter duration of intubation among patients treated with low-dose opioid anesthetics.[26,35–39] Subsequent Cochrane reviews found an earlier time to extubation and a decrease in ICU length of stay.[40,41] ICU readmission rates were found 28% lower in fast-track patients compared with conventionally treated patients.[42]

Comparisons between postoperative pulmonary function in the 2 groups demonstrated similar postoperative mechanics and rates of pulmonary complications.[36,43] Overall, fewer cardiopulmonary complications were observed among early extubation patients.[44] Pain levels between early extubated and conventionally extubated patients were also found to be similar.[45]

Additionally, no difference in cognitive functioning was found between the 2 groups.[46] Cheng noted however, that patients who received early extubation demonstrated better scores on Mini-Mental status Examinations and returned to baseline mental status earlier than patients treated with traditional postoperative care.[30] Early extubation did facilitate earlier mobilization and contributed to earlier ICU discharge.[46]

Box 6
Postoperative cardiac ICU costs

- 45% to 50% of expenses allocated to nursing staff
- 22% to 25% supportive services, such as pharmacy and respiratory therapists
- 15% to 20% supplies and equipment
- 4% to 13% medications

Data from Cheng DC, Sherry KM. Intensive care rounds: cost in the intensive care unit. London: The Medicine Group Ltd; 1996.

Direct fast track to postoperative care in the postanesthesia care unit (PACU) is also a possibility.[47] In one study, patients randomized to care in the PACU had significantly decreased time to extubation compared with the ICU, with lower rates of reintubation and complications. Median length of stay in the PACU versus the ICU was 3.3 hours versus 17.9 hours.[48]

Savings incurred from fast-track pathways stemmed from decreased use of ICU resources. Early extubation and decreased ICU length of stay shifts expenses from costly ICU admissions to the less expensive medical ward. Cheng and colleagues[25] performed the first cost comparison between a fast-track pathway (ie, extubation within 6 hours postoperatively) with a conventional management course (ie, extubation within 12–22 hours postoperatively). A fast-track pathway decreased CV ICU costs by 53% and total CABG surgical cost by 25% compared with late extubation. The savings are generated mainly from decreased ICU stay and decreased ICU nursing costs; however, surgical ward costs also decreased.[39] Total cost savings for each CABG surgery was $1699 (9%) in the early group. Savings in each department amounted to 23% in the CV ICU, 11% in the surgical wards, and 12% in respiratory therapy.[25] Decreased operating room cancellation rate was demonstrated and an increased number of procedures were able to be performed under the early extubation pathway.[25,35] At 1-year follow-up, fast-track patients were noted to use significantly fewer resources due to decreased rates of rehabilitation admission and length of stay.[42]

In a single-institution study at the Boston Medical Center, discharge data were observed between 2 periods, 1 prior to the institution of same-day admission for fast-track cardiac surgery (1990) and a period after the establishment of these protocols (1998). The introduction of these protocols reduced the mean hospital length of stay from 9.2 days to 5.4 days between 1990 and 1998. Despite a sicker patient population who required more urgent and complicated surgeries, patients who had surgery after establishment of these pathways were discharged an average of 3.8 days sooner than their prior cohorts.[38]

Reducing the duration of postoperative ventilation begins with judicious intraoperative management and physicians comfortable with airway management to advocate for early extubation. Anesthesiologists are the natural advocates for fast tracking. The evidence demonstrates the benefits to both the patients and hospital system with successful fast tracking. The next section of this article examines delirium management, another challenge of critical care medicine that has profound short-term and long-term effects for patients and poses a heavy economic burden to hospitals.

DELIRIUM: ASSOCIATED COSTS, RISK FACTORS, AND TREATMENT

Recent focus on critical care management has increasingly looked at delirium and sedation management as areas for improvement. Advances in understanding the pathophysiology of dysfunctional organs and concomitant innovations to support organ failure have improved mortality for some conditions (septic shock, stroke, myocardial infarction, and so forth) while increasing the total cost of care. Delirium—a form of acute brain dysfunction often seen in the ICU—was once viewed as a benign iatrogenic consequence of critical illness.[49] Recent investigations have radically changed historical perceptions of delirium, demonstrating poor prognosis in the long term and carrying cumulative risks rivaling other iatrogenic events.

ICU delirium is predictive of a 3-fold higher reintubation rate and greater than 10 additional hospitalization days.[50,51] Each additional day spent in delirium is associated with a 20% increased risk of prolonged hospitalization and a 10% increased risk of death. Even after controlling for preexisting comorbidities, severity of illness scores,

CV ICU Interdisciplinary Rapid Extubation Protocol (I•REP)

Place Patient Label Here

Upon ICU Admission
1. Vent settings: SIMV, RR 16, Vt 6–7.5 mL/kg of PBW, PSV10, PEEP 5, FiO_2 60% or FiO_2 specified by OR team.
2. Connect pulse oximetry and $ETCO_2$ and note values.
3. Wean FiO_2 over 5 min to maintain SpO_2 >92%.
4. At bedside OR handoff, confirm and record:
   A. Is patient a candidate for I-REP?
   B. Normal or difficult airway?
   C. Does patient have history of OSA?
5. Draw & analyze ABG after 20 min of stable vent settings. Correlate $ETCO_2$ and SpO_2 with ABG results. If patient has HCO_3 less than 18 and pH less than 7.32, repeat ABG within 1 hour. If acidemia remains, contact ICU team before vent weaning.
6. Adjust set RR for initial $ETCO_2$ range of 28–35.
7. Within 1–3h, when weaning criteria are met, begin active vent weaning per protocol.
*Vent weaning should begin at the earliest possible moment when patient meets criteria, regardless of time of day.

DATE:

OR EXIT TIME

ICU ADMISSION TIME

Admission Handoff Questions (Circle Response)

1. Is Patient a candidate for I-REP?   YES / NO

2. Normal of difficult airway?   Normal / Difficult

3. History of OSA?   YES / NO

Vent Weaning Criteria

Begin Weaning When:
1. SpO_2 greater than 92% on FiO_2 less than 60%.
2. HCO_3 greater or equal to 18
3. PEEP less than or equal to 8 cmH2O
4. Temp greater than 35 degrees C.
5. Hemodynamically stable. Pressors doses are stable or decreasing.
6. Chest tube output is stable and decreasing.
7. Patient demonstrates spontaneous respiratory efforts.
If patient is not over breathing the set RR, reduce set rate by 50% for up to 5 min to screen for presence of spontaneous respiratory efforts. RT will remain at bedside during screening.

Document Avoidable Workflow Related Delays

Extubation Criteria

1. SpO_2 greater than 92% on FiO_2 less than or equal to 50%
2. $ETCO_2$ stable and within baseline +/- 10%
3. pH >7.30
4. PS of 10 or less. PEEP 5.
5. Normal, comfortable breathing pattern. RSBI<100.
6. Patient follows instructions
7. Normal (low risk) airway as documented in the Anesthesia Record.
8. RT/RN both are in agreement to extubate.

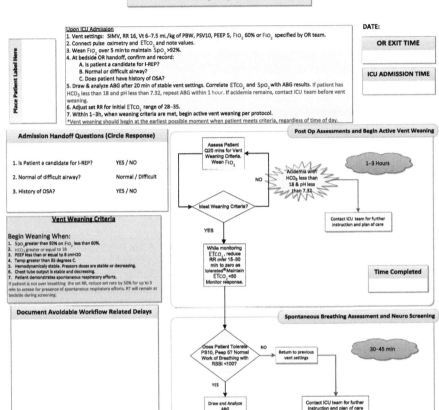

Post Op Assessments and Begin Active Vent Weaning

Assess Patient Q20 mins for Vent Weaning Criteria. Wean FiO_2

1–3 Hours

Acidemia with HCO_3 less than 18 & pH less than 7.32 → NO

Meet Weaning Criteria? → YES

Contact ICU team for further instruction and plan of care

While monitoring $ETCO_2$, reduce RR over 15–30 min to zero as tolerated* Maintain $ETCO_2$ <50 Monitor response.

Time Completed

Spontaneous Breathing Assessment and Neuro Screening

Does Patient Tolerate PS10, Peep 5? Normal Work of Breathing with RSBI <100? → NO → Return to previous vent settings

30–45 min

→ YES

Draw and Analyze ABG

Contact ICU team for further instruction and plan of care

Reassess Q15 min → NO

Can patient follow commands? Squeeze hand & lift head off pillow? → After 3 No Cycles

Time Completed

→ YES

Extubation & Post Extubation O2/Support

Meet Extubation Criteria? → NO → Contact MD for extubation instructions and plan of care

30 min

→ YES

Inform MD of plan to extubate. (Courtesy Call) → STOP

RT to extubate with RN at bedside. O2 NC or CPAP/BiPAP[b]

Time Extubated

*Ok to extubate on decreasing or stable levels of dexmedtomidine infusion

> **Box 7**
> **Early extubation after cardiac surgery**
>
> - Allows for earlier mobility
> - Decreased risk of infections and thrombosis
> - Earlier chest tube removal
> - Earlier oral intake
> - Earlier discharge from the ICU and from the hospital

coma, and the use of sedatives and analgesics, patients with ICU delirium have a more than 3-fold increased risk of 6-month mortality compared with those without delirium.[51] Up to 70% of intubated patients in the ICU develop delirium. Elderly patients receiving mechanical ventilation and requiring sedation are at the highest risk.[52]

Delirium costs $164 billion a year in the United States.[53] Compared with estimates for other conditions, including diabetes mellitus ($91.8 billion), the economic burden of delirium is substantial and noteworthy.[54] The high cost of delirium has been attributed to its impact in hospital length of stay as well as increased risk of major complications, increased use of postacute facilities, and poor functional recovery.[55,56] In the ICU, delirium is independently associated with higher ICU costs ($22,346 vs $13,332, respectively) and hospital costs ($41,836 vs $27,106, respectively) compared with those without delirium.[57] The associated annual cost of ICU delirium can be alarming. In 1 study, delirium occurred in as many as 80% of mechanically ventilated patients and was associated with and incremental increase in ICU costs of $9014 per patient.[57] Using the annual number of ICU admissions for respiratory failure requiring mechanical ventilation as an estimate (approximately 880,000–2,760,000), the cost increase associated with delirium in just in the ICU can range between $6.5 billion and $20.4 billion.[57–59]

Approximately 30% to 40% of the cases of delirium are thought to be preventable, making delirium an appealing target for interventions to prevent associated complications and costs.[60] In an executive summary published by the American Association of Retired Persons (AARP), the Harvard School of Medicine and Harvard School of Public Health, delirium was considered 1 of the 6 leading causes of preventable injury in those greater than 65 years old.[61] It is often considered a quality indicator for health care provided to elderly patients.[60,62] Efforts at monitoring and treating hospital-acquired delirium have improved outcomes in not only mortality but also ICU and hospital length of stay.

◀──────────────────────────────

Fig. 5. Example of a CV ICU interdisciplinary rapid extubation protocol. ABG, arterial blood gas; Bipap, Bilevel positive airway pressure; CPAP, continuous positive airway pressure; ETCO2, end tidal carbon dioxide; FiO2, Fraction of inspired Oxygen; HCO3, bicarbonate levels; MD, medical doctor; NC, nasal cannula; OR, operating room; OSA, obstructive sleep apnea; PBW, predicted body weight; PEEP, Positive End Expiratory Pressure; PS, pressure support; PSV, Pressure support ventilation; RN, registered nurse; RR, respiratory rate; RSBI, rapid shallow breathing index; RT, respiratory therapist; SIMV, synchronized intermittent mandatory ventilation; SPO2, oxygenation saturation; Vent, ventilator; Vt, tidal volume. [a] When rate is zero, patient will be on PSV 10, PEEP 5 – supported spontaneous breathing. [b] If patient is morbidly obese or has history of obstructive sleep apnea (OSA), extubate to CPAP of 8 to 10 cm or BiPAP 10/5 of H_2O for 2 hours. Titrate pressure to alleviate any observed upper airway obstruction and for patient comfort.

Inouye and colleagues[60] used a multicomponent intervention aimed at mitigating delirium and found that with a total cost $139,506, 22 cases of delirium were prevented when compared with the group receiving usual care (**Boxes 8** and **9**).

Of the many clinical interventions known to predispose for delirium, no intervention has been more implicated and studied than the use and choice of sedative/analgesic agents. Providing sedation for patient comfort is an integral component of bedside ICU care. Targeted sedation for a calm, pain-free, and interactive patient remains a main goal. Evidence-based guidelines for this are continually updated to improve outcomes (**Fig. 6**).[63]

The use of benzodiazepines, such as lorazepam and midazolam, has been strongly associated with the development of delirium.[64,65] These agents work as agonists at the γ-aminobutyric acid receptor, resulting in a decreased level of consciousness and impaired sleep. Novel agents, such as the α_2-receptor agonists (ie, dexmedetomidine), may reduce the prevalence and duration of delirium.[66,67] Protocols that routinely minimize sedation and regularly assess a patient's readiness for extubation improve outcomes.[68,69]

These protocols along with the daily monitoring of delirium using the Confusion Assessment Method for the ICU (CAM-ICU) screen and the implementation of early mobility form what are called the ABCDE bundle:

- Awakening and breathing coordination
- Delirium monitoring and management
- Early exercise/mobility

This bundle's goal is to liberate and animate ICU patients requiring mechanical ventilation. This can reduce the burden of ICU-acquired disorders, such as weakness and delirium (**Box 10**).[70]

The adoption of the ABCDE bundle in a mixed critically ill patient population is effective and safe and can decrease the length of mechanical ventilation by as much as 3 days.[75] Cost savings from adoption of such protocols have been estimated to range from $860 to nearly $6000 per patient, amounting to a decrease in ICU costs by 35% and ward costs by 30%.[76,77]

Each part of the bundle requires the collaboration of an interdisciplinary team consisting of physicians, nurses, physical therapists, and respiratory therapists who work synergistically to minimize sedation, perform breathing trials in awake patients, and mobilize patients who can participate with therapy. ICUs must strive to monitor their adherence to spontaneous awakening trials (SATs)/spontaneous breathing trials (SBTs) and to the vigilant monitoring of delirium using validated methods (CAM-ICU).

Box 8
Risk factors for delirium

- Preexisting cognitive impairment
- Elderly age
- Sleep and sensory deprivation (poor vision/poor hearing)
- Immobility
- Laboratory abnormalities (hyponatremia, azotemia, hypocalcemia, etc.)
- Infection
- Use of restraints and catheters

Box 9
Behavioral interventions to reduce delirium

- Repeated reorientation
- Nonpharmacologic sleep hygiene protocols
- Early mobilization
- Timely removal of catheters and physical restraints
- Provision of magnifying lenses and hearing aid to reconnect the patient with the environment

---

Delirium should not be thought of just as a hospital problem or a complication. Recent evidence suggests that long-term cognitive impairment persists well after ICU and hospital discharge for both old and young patients who develop delirium during their critical illness. At 12 months after discharge, approximately 1 in 3 patients has global cognition and executive function scores similar to patients with moderate traumatic brain injury; approximately 1 in 4 has scores similar to patients with mild

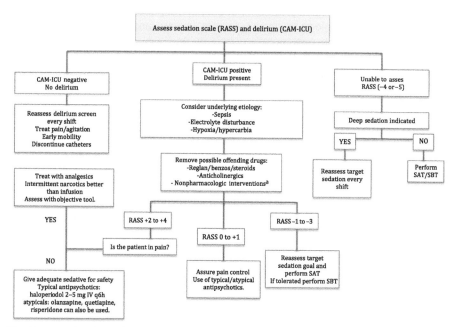

Fig. 6. Example of a delirium assessment and sedation weaning protocol. SAT, minimize or stop sedation to awaken patient. SBT, CPAP/ATC trial if on 50% and less than PEEP 8 and SATs greater than 90%. [a] Nonpharmacologic interventions: provide visual/hearing aids, reorient patient repetitively, include familiar objects from home in daily care (painting, picture, object etc.), allow daily activity, ambulate if able, nonverbal music, maximize sleep hygiene, lights off at night, on during day, and control excess noise at night. ATC, automatic tube compensation; benzos, benzodiazepines; CPAP, continuous positive airway pressure; PEEP, positive end expiratory pressure; RASS, Richmond Agitation-Sedation Scale. (*Adapted from* Pun B, Ely EW. The importance of diagnosing and managing ICU delirium. Chest 2007;132:633.)

Box 10
Definitions

- Liberation refers to reducing the need for mechanical ventilation through the use of coordinated SATs[2] and SBTs—"awake the patient so the patient can breathe."[71,72]

- Animation refers to early mobilization to mitigate the development of ICU delirium and other ICU acquired disorders, such as weakness.[73,74]

Data from Refs.[2,71-74]

Alzheimer disease.[78] A longer duration of delirium was associated with worse long-term global cognition, an association that was independent of sedatives used. The true societal cost from hospital-acquired delirium remains to be evaluated, with the potential of becoming a growing public health problem given the large number of patients treated in ICUs.

FUTURE CONSIDERATIONS

Equipped with the tools of the modern ICU, intensivists will continue to rescue and sustain life even in the most severely ill patients. Many current ICUs and CV ICUs are staffed by anesthesiology-trained intensivists who are familiar with both intraoperative anesthetic use and postoperative sedation and ventilator management. This positions anesthesiologists to be strong advocates for enacting both fast-track pathways for cardiac patients and sedation weaning and delirium protocols for all critically ill patients. Even for nonintensivists, the use of anesthetics and providing anesthetic care in a way that sets patients up for early extubation are ways that such pathways can be facilitated. Direct conversations with surgeons in the operating room should be prompted to discuss feasibility of early extubation for each patient depending on preoperative and intraoperative factors. The economic impact of early extubation, sedation, and delirium prevention and management are significant and it is only a matter of time before efforts cross institutional silos and enter a larger national discussion.

Increasing health care costs necessitate a change in current practice to a value- and cost-focused model. Critical care costs and outcomes are going to be increasingly scrutinized in the new cost-conscious health care world. With the current focus of expanding anesthetic care beyond the realms of the operating room, these pathways provide a means for anesthesiologists to provide the best value-based care in the postoperative and ICU environments. This will provide the key to future extensions of the anesthesia specialty and providing true value-based anesthetic care throughout all aspects of patient care.

REFERENCES

1. National Health Expenditures 2013 Highlights.
2. Cosgrove T. Value-based health care is inevitable and that's good. Harv Bus Rev 2013.
3. Brill S. What I learned from my $190,000 open-heart surgery. Time 2015;185: 34–44.
4. Deloitte. The hidden costs of US healthcare.
5. McKinsey Global Institute. Accounting for the Cost of Health Care in the United States. 2007.

6. Lazard Asset Management. US equity: performance summary as of December 31, 2012. 2013.
7. Mullins PM, Goyal M, Pines JM. National growth in intensive care unit admissions from emergency departments in the United States from 2002 to 2009. Acad Emerg Med 2013;20(5):479–86.
8. Utilization of Intensive Care Services, 2011. Healthcare Cost and Utilization Project.
9. Gooch RA, Kahn JM. ICU bed supply, utilization, and health care spending: an example of demand elasticity. JAMA 2014;311:567–8.
10. Wunsch H, Angus DC, Harrison DA, et al. Comparison of medical admissions to intensive care units in the United States and United Kingdom. Am J Respir Crit Care Med 2011;183:1666–73.
11. Esserman L, Belkora J, Lenert L. Potentially ineffective care: a new outcome to assess the limits of critical care. JAMA 1995;274:1544–51.
12. Noseworthy TW, Konopad E, Shustack A, et al. Cost accounting of adult intensive care: methods and human and capital inputs. Crit Care Med 1996;24:1168–72.
13. Dasta JF, McLaughlin TP, Mody SH, et al. Daily cost of an intensive care unit day: the contribution of mechanical ventilation. Crit Care Med 2005;33:1266–71.
14. Porter M, Olmsted Teisberg E. Redefining healthcare. Creating value-based competition on results. Watertown (MA): Harvard Business Review Press; 2006.
15. PriceWaterhouseCoopers Health Research Institute. The price of excess: identifying waste in healthcare spending. 2008.
16. Skinner J, Fisher E. Reflections on variation. The Dartmouth Atlas of Health Care; 2010. Available at: http://www.dartmouthatlas.org/downloads/press/Skinner_Fisher_DA_05_10.pdf.
17. Rand Corporation. The First National Report Card on Quality of Healthcare Care in America. Research Highlights.
18. Guo C, Macario A. Financial and operational analysis for non-operating room anesthesia.
19. Macario A. What does one minute of operating room time cost? J Clin Anesth 2010;22(4):233–6.
20. American Heart Association. Heart disease & stroke statistics. Our guide to current statistics and the supplement our heart & stroke facts. 2009 Update At-A-Glance.
21. National Institutes of Health. National Heart, Lung, and Blood Institute. Fact book fiscal year 2009.
22. Inpatient Surgery FastStats. CDC/National Center for Health Statistics. Available at: http://www.cdc.gov/nchs/fastats/inpatient-surgery.htm. Accessed December 14, 2014.
23. Characteristics of operating room procedures in U.S. Hospitals, 2011. Healthcare Cost and Utilization Project.
24. CMS Inpatient Charge Data FY 2012. Available at: http://www.cms.gov/Research-Statistics-Data-and-Systems/Statistics-Trends-and-Reports/Medicare-Provider-Charge-Data/Inpatient2012.html. Accessed December 14, 2014.
25. Cheng DC, Karski J, Peniston C, et al. Early tracheal extubation after coronary artery bypass graft surgery reduces costs and improves resource use. A prospective, randomized, controlled trial. Anesthesiology 1996;85:1300–10.
26. Myles PS, Daly DJ, Djaiani G, et al. A systematic review of the safety and effectiveness of fast-track cardiac anesthesia. Anesthesiology 2003;99:982–7.
27. Hamilton A, Norris C, Wensel R. Cost reduction in cardiac surgery. Can J Cardiol 1994;10:721–7.

28. Taylor GJ, Mikell FL, Moses HW. Determinants of hospital charges for coronary artery bypass surgery: the economic consequences of postoperative complications. Am J Cardiol 1990;65:309–13.

29. Weintraub WS, Jones EL, Craver J. Determinants of prolonged length of hospital stay after coronary bypass surgery. Circulation 1989;80:276–84.

30. Cheng DC. Fast-track cardiac surgery: economic implications in postoperative care. J Cardiothorac Vasc Anesth 1998;12:72–9.

31. Cowper PA, DeLong ER, Peterson ED, et al. Variability in cost of coronary bypass surgery in New York State: potential for cost savings. Am Heart J 2002;143: 130–9.

32. Ghali WA, Hall RE, Ash AS, et al. Identifying pre- and postoperative predictors of cost and length of stay for coronary artery bypass surgery. Am J Med Qual 1999; 14:248–54.

33. Silbert BS, Myles PS. Is fast-track cardiac anesthesia now the global standard of care? Anesth Analg 2009;108:689–91.

34. Cheng DC. Fast track cardiac surgery pathways: early extubation, process of care, and cost containment. Anesthesiology 1998;88:1429–33.

35. Michalopoulos A, Nikolaides C, Antzaka C, et al. Change in anaesthesia practice and postoperative sedation shortens ICU and hospital length of stay following coronary artery bypass surgery. Respir Med 1998;92(8):1066–70.

36. Cheng DC, Karski J, Peniston C, et al. Morbidity outcome in early versus conventional tracheal extubation after coronary artery bypass grafting: a prospective randomized controlled trial. J Thorac Cardiovasc Surg 1996;112(3):755–64.

37. Reyes A, Vega G, Blancas R, et al. Early vs conventional extubation after cardiac surgery with cardiopulmonary bypass. Chest 1997;112(1):193–201.

38. Lazar HL, Fitzgerald C, Ahmad T, et al. Early discharge after coronary artery bypass graft surgery: are patients really going home earlier? J Thorac Cardiovasc Surg 2001;121:943–50.

39. van Mastrigt GA, Heijmans J, Severens JL, et al. Short-stay intensive care after coronary artery bypass surgery: randomized clinical trial on safety and cost-effectiveness. Crit Care Med 2006;34(1):65–75.

40. Zhu F, Lee A, Chee YE. Fast-track cardiac care for adult cardiac surgical patients. Cochrane Database Syst Rev 2012;(10):CD003587.

41. Hawkes CA, Dhileepan S, Foxcroft D. Early extubation for adult cardiac surgical patients. Cochrane Database Syst Rev 2003;(4):CD003587.

42. Cheng DC, Wall C, Djaiani G, et al. Randomized assessment of resource use in fast-track cardiac surgery 1-year after hospital discharge. Anesthesiology 2003; 98(3):651–7.

43. Nicholson DJ, Kowalski SE, Hamilton GA, et al. Postoperative pulmonary function in coronary artery bypass graft surgery patients undergoing early tracheal extubation: a comparison between short-term mechanical ventilation and early extubation. J Cardiothorac Vasc Anesth 2002;16(1):27–31.

44. Quasha AL, Loeber N, Feeley TW, et al. Postoperative respiratory care: a controlled trial of early and late extubation following coronary artery bypass grafting. Anesthesiology 1980;52(2):135–41.

45. Pettersson PH, Settergren G, Owall A. Similar pain scores after early and late extubation in heart surgery with cardiopulmonary bypass. J Cardiothorac Vasc Anesth 2004;18(1):64–7.

46. Dumas A, Dupuis GH, Searle N, et al. Early versus late extubation after coronary artery bypass grafting: effects on cognitive function. J Cardiothorac Vasc Anesth 1999;13(2):130–5.

47. Probst S, Cech C, Haentschel D, et al. A specialized post anaesthetic care unit improves fast-track management in cardiac surgery: a prospective randomized trial. Crit Care 2014;18(4):468.

48. Flynn M, Reddy S, Shepherd W, et al. Fast-tracking revisited: routine cardiac surgical patients need minimal intensive care. Eur J Cardiothorac Surg 2004;25:116–22.

49. Ely EW, Stephens RK, Jackson JC, et al. Current opinions regarding the importance, diagnosis, and management of delirium in the intensive care unit: a survey of 912 healthcare professionals. Am J Respir Crit Care Med 2002;167:969.

50. Ely EW, Gautam S, Margolin R, et al. The impact of delirium in the intensive care unit on hospital length of stay. Intensive Care Med 2001;27:1892–900.

51. Miller RR, Shintani A, Girard TD, et al. Delirium predicts extubation failure [abstract]. Proc Am Thorac Soc 2006;3:42.

52. McNicoll L, Pisani MA, Zhang Y, et al. Delirium in the intensive care unit: occurrence and clinical course in older patients. J Am Geriatr Soc 2003;51(5):591.

53. Leslie DL, Marcantonio ER, Zhang Y, et al. One-year health care costs associated with delirium in the elderly population. Arch Intern Med 2008;168:27–32.

54. Hogan P, Dall T, Nikolov P. Economic costs of diabetes in the US in 2002. Diabetes Care 2003;26(3):917–32.

55. Thomas RI, Cameron DJ, Fahs MC. A prospective study of delirium and prolonged hospital stay. Arch Gen Psychiatry 1988;45:937–40.

56. Francis J, Kapoor WN. Prognosis after hospital discharge of older medical patients with delirium. J Am Geriatr Soc 1992;40:601–6.

57. Milbrandt EB, Deppen S, Harrison PL, et al. Costs associated with delirium in mechanically ventilated patients. Crit Care Med 2004;32:955–62.

58. Vincent JL, Akca S, De Mendonca A, et al. The epidemiology of acute respiratory failure in critically ill patients. Chest 2002;121:1602–9.

59. Dennett SL, Zeiher BG, Bowman L, et al. Who receives mechanical ventilation in the U. S.: diagnoses and resource use. Crit Care Med 2003;30:A128.

60. Inouye SK, Bogardus ST Jr, Charpentier PA, et al. A multicomponent intervention to prevent delirium in hospitalized older patients. N Engl J Med 1999;340(9):669.

61. Rothschild JM, Leape LL. The nature and extent of medical injury in older patients: research report. September 2000. AARP Public Policy Institute Issue Paper 2000–17. Available at: http://assets.aarp.org/rgcenter/health/2000_17_injury.pdf. Accessed March 25, 2007.

62. Agency for Healthcare Research and Quality (AHRQ). National quality clearinghouse measure: delirium: proportion of patients meeting diagnostic criteria on the confusion assessment method (CAM). Available at: http://www.qualitymeasures. ahrq.gov/content. aspx?id=27635. Accessed January 3, 2013.

63. Barr J, Fraser GL, Puntillo K, et al. Clinical practice guidelines for the management of pain, agitation, and delirium in adult patients in the intensive care unit. Crit Care Med 2013;41(1):263–306.

64. Pandharipande PP, Shintani A, Peterson J, et al. Lorazepam is an independent risk factor for transitioning to delirium in intensive care unit patients. Anesthesiology 2006;104:21–6.

65. Dubois MJ, Bergeron N, Dumont M, et al. Delirium in an intensive care unit: a study of risk factors. Intensive Care Med 2001;27:1297–304.

66. Maldonado JR, van der Starre PJ, Wysong A. Post-operative sedation and the incidence of ICU delirium in cardiac surgery patients [abstract]. Anesthesiology 2003;99:A465.

67. Pandharipande PP, Pun BT, Herr DL, et al. Effect of sedation with dexmedetomidine vs lorazepam on acute brain dys- function in mechanically ventilated patients: the MENDS randomized controlled trial. JAMA 2007;298:2644–53.

68. Girard TD, Kress JP, Fucks BD, et al. Efficacy and safety of a paired sedation and ventilator weaning protocol for mechanically ventilated patients in intensive care (Awakening and Breathing Controlled trial): a randomized controlled trial. Lancet 2008;371:126–34.

69. Strom T, Martinussen T, Toft P. A protocol of no sedation for critically ill patients receiving mechanical ventilation: a randomized trial. Lancet 2010;375:475–80.

70. Vasilevskis EE, Ely EW, Speroff T, et al. Reducing iatrogenic risks: ICU-acquired delirium and weakness—Crossing the quality chasm. Chest 2010;138:1224–33.

71. Kress JP, Pohlman AS, O'Connor MF, et al. Daily interruption of sedative infusions in critically ill patients undergoing mechanical ventila- tion. N Engl J Med 2000; 342:1471–7.

72. Ely EW, Baker AM, Dunagan DP, et al. Effect on the duration of mechanical venti- lation of identifying patients capable of breathing spontaneously. N Engl J Med 1996;335:1864–9.

73. Schweickert WD, Pohlman MC, Pohlman AS, et al. Early physical and occupational therapy in mechanically ventilated, critically ill patients: a randomised controlled trial. Lancet 2009;373:1874–82.

74. Needham DM. Mobilizing patients in the intensive care unit: improving neuromus- cular weakness and physical function. JAMA 2008;300:1685–90.

75. Balas M, Vasilevskis EE, Olsen KM, et al. Effectiveness and safety of the awakening and breathing coordination, delirium monitoring/management, andearly exercise/ mobility bundle. Crit Care Med 2014;42(5):1024–36.

76. Awissi DK, Bégin C, Moisan J, et al. I-SAVE study: impact of sedation, analgesia, and delirium protocols evaluated in the intensive care unit: an economic evalua- tion. Ann Pharmacother 2012;46:21–8.

77. Shorr A, Micek ST, Jackson WL. Economic implications of an evidence-based sepsis protocol: can we improve outcomes and lower costs? Crit Care Med 2007;35:1257–62.

78. Pandharipande PP, Girard TD, Jackson JK, et al. Long-term cognitive impairment after critical illness. N Engl J Med 2013;369(14):1306–16.

Perioperative Surgical Home: Perspective II

Thomas R. Vetter, MD, MPH[a],*, Keith A. Jones, MD[b]

KEYWORDS

- Perioperative surgical home • Value-based care • Value stream map
- Personalized care • Population health management • Health care informatics
- Health care analytics • Clinical decision support

KEY POINTS

- The Perioperative Surgical Home emphasizes the standardization, coordination, transitions, and value of care, throughout the perioperative continuum, including during the post-hospital discharge phase.
- Current and imminent fundamental changes in governmental and commercial reimbursement models are creating a "burning platform" for concordant obligatory changes in perioperative health care delivery.
- The Perioperative Surgical Home can achieve all 3 elements of the Institute for Healthcare Improvement Triple Aim: (1) optimizing the individual experience of care, (2) improving the health of populations, and (3) reducing per capita costs of care.
- The Perioperative Surgical Home is an innovative Lean method application, which can be detailed as a value stream process activity map, which includes all 4 phases of patient care and the respective multiple patient contact points.
- Health care informatics, analytics, and decision support are fundamental mechanisms for achieving the practice change in management that is required for the Perioperative Surgical Home to implement and sustain quality, safety, and satisfaction improvement, and cost-reduction strategies, to thus maximize value-based care.

Every few years we stop and analyze where we are today and what the gaps are we have to fill, and right now we are on the next cusp in health care with work to do on safety, patient flow, efficiency, and on getting the right care to the right patient at the right time and place.
— *Maureen Bisognano, President and CEO, Institute for Healthcare Improvement.*

Funding: UAB Department of Anesthesiology and Perioperative Medicine internal funds.
Commercial or Financial Conflicts of Interest: None reported by T.R. Vetter or K.A. Jones.
[a] Department of Anesthesiology and Perioperative Medicine, University of Alabama at Birmingham, JT862, 619 19th Street South, Birmingham, AL 35249, USA; [b] Department of Anesthesiology and Perioperative Medicine, University of Alabama at Birmingham, JT804, 619 19th Street South, Birmingham, AL 35249, USA
* Corresponding author.
E-mail address: tvetter@uab.edu

http://dx.doi.org/10.1016/j.anclin.2015.07.002
1932-2275/15/$ – see front matter © 2015 Elsevier Inc. All rights reserved.
anesthesiology.theclinics.com

INTRODUCTION

The combined effects of expanded health insurance coverage under the 2010 Patient Protection and Affordable Care Act (ACA), faster economic growth, and an aging population (the "Silver Tsunami") are expected to result in greater demand for health care goods and services in the United States between 2015 and 2023.[1] The health care share of the United States gross domestic product is thus projected to increase to 19.3% in 2023.[1]

Surgical care currently accounts for an estimated 52% of hospital admission expenses in the United States.[2] Fragmentation and inefficiencies in delivery of care, defensive medicine, discordant incentives between stakeholders who deliver versus those who pay for care, and a lack of emphasis on value are contributing to excessive surgical expenditures.[3,4]

To address these and other contributing factors, the Perioperative Surgical Home model has been developed using the guiding principles of the Patient-Centered Medical Home.[5,6] The Perioperative Surgical Home is a similarly very patient-centered approach, with an emphasis on the standardization, coordination, transitions, and value of care, throughout the perioperative continuum, including during the post-hospital discharge phase.[5] The early adopters of this new perioperative care model will be challenged to demonstrate that it actually does achieve these espoused goals. The Perioperative Surgical Home is also predicated on a robust yet often novel interdisciplinary collaboration between an institution's surgeons and its anesthesiologists, hospitalists, and intensivists.

POPULATION HEALTH MANAGEMENT

Health care delivery and payment systems in the United States must continue to be reformed to address currently untenably increasing health care expenditures while at the same time increasing the quality of care.[7] In his 2012 Shattuck lecture, Institute of Medicine (IOM) President Harvey Fineberg noted that "America's health system is neither as successful as it should be nor as sustainable as it must be."[8]

Fineberg[8] posited (**Table 1**) that a successful health system has 3 key attributes:

- Healthy people
- Superior care
- Fairness

Furthermore, he posited (see **Table 1**) that a sustainable health system has 3 key attributes:

- Affordability
- Acceptability to key constituents
- Adaptability

Fineberg[8] also observed that proposed solutions need to focus on the specific ultimate outcome of interest: the overall population's health and each individual's health.[8]

Berwick and colleagues[9] and the Institute for Healthcare Improvement (IHI) have promulgated the "Triple Aim" as a basic framework for the much needed overall health care reform in the United States.[10] The IHI Triple Aim comprises 3 interdependent goals: (1) optimizing the individual experience of care, (2) improving the health of populations, and (3) reducing per capita costs of care.[9,10]

The Perioperative Surgical Home is capable of achieving all 3 elements of the IHI Triple Aim. Furthermore, achieving the IHI Triple Aim can provide leverage for

Table 1	
Key attributes of a successful and sustainable health system	
	Definition
Successful Health System Attributes	
Healthy people	A population that attains the highest level of health possible
Superior care	Effective, safe, timely, patient-centered, equitable, and efficient
Fairness	Treatment is applied without discrimination or disparities to all individuals and families, regardless of age, group identity, or place, and that the system is fair to the health professionals, institutions, and businesses supporting and delivering care
Sustainable Health System Attributes	
Affordability	For patients and families, employers, and the government
Acceptability	To key constituents, including patients and health professionals
Adaptability	Health and health care needs are not static, so a health system must respond adaptively to new diseases, changing demographics, scientific discoveries, and dynamic technologies to remain viable

Data from Fineberg HV. Shattuck lecture. A successful and sustainable health system—how to get there from here. N Engl J Med 2012;366:1020–7.

anesthesiologists and its other advocates to obtain the needed institutional political and fiscal support for developing and implementing a Perioperative Surgical Home model.[11] The Perioperative Surgical Home seeks to improve the health of its identified target population: the progressively aging and increasingly chronically ill population undergoing surgery in the United States.[11]

The Agency for Healthcare Research and Quality (AHRQ) has defined practice-based population health management as an approach to care that uses data on a group ("population") of patients within a primary care practice or group of practices ("practice-based") to improve the care and clinical outcomes of patients within that practice.[12] The AHRQ has identified a series of 5 information management functional domains to support proactive population management (**Box 1**).[12]

Though initially applied within the context of the Patient-Centered Medical Home, the authors believe that these tenets of practice-based population health management espoused by AHRQ (especially, information technology-based identification of higher-risk patient subgroups and tracking of performance metrics relative to national guidelines or peer comparison groups) are very applicable to the congruent Perioperative Surgical Home.

"BURNING PLATFORM" OF CHANGING REIMBURSEMENT MODELS

Over the past several years, commercial payers and governmental insurance agencies in the United States have enacted measures designed to enhance the value of patient care (**Fig. 1**). Initially, these measures have included a combination of incentives and penalties designed to promote information transparency and quality reporting, utilization of clinical informatics (including fully integrated electronic health records to improve the accuracy and sharing of patient information), and adoption of well-proven processes to decrease complications and mishaps during a patient's hospitalization.

Specifically, under the provisions of the 2010 federal ACA, the United States Center for Medicare and Medicaid Services (CMS) established its Hospital Readmissions

> **Box 1**
> **Five functional domains of information management that can support proactive population management**
>
> *Domain 1: Identify subpopulations of patients.* Practices can target patients who require preventive care or tests.
>
> *Domain 2: Examine detailed characteristics of identified subpopulations.* Information management systems can allow practices to run queries to narrow down the subpopulation of patients, or to access patient records or additional patient information.
>
> *Domain 3: Create reminders for patients and providers.* Information on patients can be made actionable through notifications for patients and members of the practice.
>
> *Domain 4: Track performance measures.* Practices can gain an understanding of how they are providing care relative to national guidelines or peer comparison groups.
>
> *Domain 5: Make data available in multiple forms.* Information may be most useful to practices if it can be printed, saved, or exported and if it can be displayed graphically.
>
> *From* Cusack CM, Knudson AD, Kronstadt JL, et al. Practice-Based Population Health: Information Technology to Support Transformation to Proactive Primary Care (Prepared for the AHRQ National Resource Center for Health Information Technology under Contract No. 290-04-0016.) AHRQ Publication No. 10-0092-EF. Rockville, MD: Agency for Healthcare Research and Quality. July 2010.

Reduction Program (HRRP), which requires CMS to reduce payments to acute care hospitals with excessive readmissions beginning on October 1, 2012. For the federal fiscal year 2015, CMS has expanded the HRRP to include patients undergoing elective total hip arthroplasty and total knee arthroplasty, with a 3% maximum penalty for excessive readmissions.[13]

The ACA also established the CMS Hospital Acquired Condition (HAC) Reduction Program. A HAC is a reasonably preventable condition that a patient did not have on admission to a hospital, but which developed during the hospital stay. Hospital

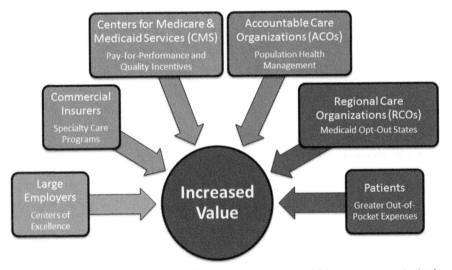

Fig. 1. Measures enacted by commercial payers and governmental insurance agencies in the United States to enhance the value of patient care.

performance under the HAC Reduction Program is determined based on a hospital's Total HAC Score, which can range from 1 to 10. The higher a hospital's Total HAC Score, the worse the hospital has performed under the HAC Reduction Program. In fiscal year 2015, the ACA requires the Secretary of the Department of Health and Human Services (DHHS) to reduce payments to hospitals that rank in the quartile of hospitals with the highest Total HAC Scores by 1%.[14]

The CMS HRRP and HAC Reduction Program are cost-neutral to the payer, as they use the reduced payments to the less compliant health care providers to reward those that have succeeded in implementing the measures.

With the CMS Hospital Value-Based Purchasing (VBP) program, these incentives and penalties have more recently transitioned from process-based to value-based measures.[15] These value measures include care delivery efficiency, which is determined by the CMS Spending per Beneficiary Measure (MSPBM).[16] The CMS MSPBM includes patient safety indicators such as the incidence of catheter-associated urinary tract infections (CAUTI) and central line–associated bloodstream infections (CLABSI), and mortality from congestive heart failure. As of October 1, 2014, CMS began using the AHRQ Patient Safety for Selected Indicators (PSI-90 composite) as its core metric in its pay-for-performance HAC Reduction program and the Hospital VBP program.[17]

Even more challenging and transformative for health care providers, payers are now moving to value-based payment models designed to substantially promote hospital and physician accountability for meeting current and future value measures. At their core, these payment models increase the financial risk ("accountability") to providers to consistently deliver high-value care to defined populations. These changes are expected to progress rapidly in the United States by way of the Accountable Care Organization (ACO) model set forth in the 2010 ACA.[18] To this end, the first 32 Medicare ACOs (the so-called pioneer ACOs) were announced in late 2011.[19] By early 2014 the number of ACOs nationwide had increased to more than 600, and the total number of estimated covered lives in public and private ACOs has risen to 18.2 million.[20] Furthermore, regional care organizations, with substantial provider-shared financial risk, have been created in some states (eg, Alabama) that opted out of the Medicaid expansion provision of the 2010 ACA.

The announced goal of the DHHS is to increase the proportion of federal payments related to value to 30% by the end of 2016 and to 50% by the end of 2018. The Health Care Transformation Task Force, a coalition of several of the country's largest health care systems and commercial insurers, has proposed an initiative to transition the way providers and hospitals are paid from the traditional volume-based, fee-for-service contracts to one predominately linked to the value of the care. The expressed commitment of this task force is to shift the bulk of nongovernmental health care payments to a value-based arrangement by 2020.

Finally, in part as a consequence of the required increase in information transparency and quality reporting by hospitals and health systems, consumers, including individual patients and businesses, are now choosing to preferentially obtain certain traditionally high-cost subspecialty services at the highest-quality programs (ie, centers of excellence). For example, Lowes has contracted with Cleveland Clinic for heart surgery, General Electric with Northwestern Memorial Hospital for total joint replacement surgery, and Walmart with several health care systems to provide transplants, heart surgery, and spine surgery. In a more sweeping initiative, in 2014 Boeing entered into a shared saving program with University of Washington Medicine and Providence Health & Services for health care services for its 27,000 employees.

WHAT IS VALUE IN HEALTH CARE?

Porter posed the salient question, "What is value in health care?" and in turn defined it as the health outcomes achieved per dollar spent.[21,22] Porter observed that value in health care remains largely unmeasured and misunderstood, in part because its "stakeholders have myriad, often conflicting goals, including access to services, profitability, high quality, cost containment, safety, convenience, patient-centeredness, and satisfaction."[21] In the resulting contentious health care environment, all its stakeholders nevertheless may embrace a value framework, given its unifying primary goal of improving outcomes and doing so as efficiently as possible.[23]

As noted earlier, the development of the Perioperative Surgical Home has been guided by the principles of the primary care–focused Patient-Centered Medical Home.[5,6] Health care, and its attendant value, are ultimately patient centered. Both of these new models of care should thus seek "to improve value for patients, where value is [specifically] defined as *patient outcomes* achieved relative to the amount of money spent."[24] This translates into a health care value equation for the Perioperative Surgical Home (**Fig. 2**), whose numerator includes:

Quality
- Quality of postoperative recovery, including pain intensity, nausea/vomiting, delirium
- Functional status, including activities of daily living
- Health-related quality of life
- Clinician adherence to evidence-based best practices
- Rate of surgical case delays and cancellations on day of surgery
- Acute hospital length of stay
- Post-hospital discharge length of stay in a skilled nursing facility
- Hospital readmission rate after discharge home or to a skilled nursing facility

Safety
- Perioperative mortality
- Perioperative complications
- Postoperative failure-to-rescue
- Intensive care unit admission and readmission rates
- Blood transfusion rate

Satisfaction
- Patient-reported
- Family and other caregiver-reported
- Clinician-reported

Many of these elements have fiscal ramifications for providers, including financial incentives and penalties based on achieving external benchmarks. These various domains and metrics should be measured in the intraoperative and immediate postoperative periods and during at least the 30 days after hospital discharge.[25] The satisfaction domain should also assess the patient's perspective on the efficiency

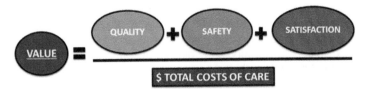

Fig. 2. Health care value equation for the Perioperative Surgical Home model.

or "patient-centric ergonomics" of the delivered perioperative care. The total costs of care in the denominator of the health care value equation (see **Fig. 2**) should include not only conventional direct medical costs but also, whenever possible, indirect medical costs (eg, lost productivity and wages of the patient and family caregivers).

STRATEGIES TO INCREASE THE VALUE OF CARE PROVIDED BY THE PERIOPERATIVE SURGICAL HOME

Top-down insights into the health care value proposition can be gained from a 2012 IOM Roundtable on Value & Science-Driven Health Care, which generated "A CEO Checklist for high-value health care"[26] that included 10 salient items (**Box 2**).

As stated by the roundtable's chief executive officer participants, "The Checklist's 10 items reflect the strategies that, in our experiences and those of others, have proven effective and essential to improving quality and reducing costs."[26] Several of the provided tangible examples of these checklist items are noteworthy in their delivery of improved value of perioperative care.

Evidence-based care protocols, which are preferably developed and refined within an institution based on local issues and circumstances, improve the reproducibility and standardization of care.[26] The cardiac surgeons at Geisinger Health System thus applied evidence or consensus best practices in creating standardized order sets, decision-support tools, and reminders in their electronic medical record for elective coronary artery bypass grafting. This effort resulted in a 67% reduction in operative mortality, a 1.3-day decrease in length of stay, and a nearly 5% decreased cost per case.[26]

Real patient-centered care is predicated on shared patient-clinician decision making and patient-clinician collaboration on care plans.[26] The Cleveland Clinic

---

Box 2
A chief executive officer (CEO) checklist for high-value health care

Foundational Elements

- Governance priority: visible and determined leadership by CEO and Board
- Culture of continuous improvement: commitment to ongoing, real-time learning

Infrastructure Fundamentals

- Information technology best practices: automated, reliable information to and from the point of care
- Evidence protocols: effective, efficient, and consistent care
- Resource utilization: optimized use of personnel, physical space, and other resources

Care Delivery Priorities

- Integrated care: right care, right setting, right providers, right teamwork
- Shared decision making: patient-clinician collaboration on care plans
- Targeted services: tailored community and clinic interventions for resource-intensive patients

Reliability and Feedback

- Embedded safeguards: supports and prompts to reduce injury and infection
- Internal transparency: visible progress in performance, outcomes, and costs

From Cosgrove D, Fisher M, Gabow P, et al. A CEO checklist for high-value health care. Washington, DC: Institute of Medicine; 2012. Reprinted with permission from the National Academy of Sciences, Courtesy of the National Academies Press, Washington, DC.

thus implemented a process in lung transplant patients whereby daily "huddles" were held with the patient, family members, and all caregivers regarding expected progress and a consistent plan. This effort resulted in 1.5-day decrease in length of stay, a 3% improvement in 30-day survival, a 28% improvement in patient satisfaction, and a 6% decrease in total cost of care.[26]

Variability in clinician practice is inevitable. However, providing clinicians with transparent, granular data about their practice variability, performance in comparison with internal and external benchmarks, and resource utilization and attendant costs can guide them to deliver improved value.[26] The Cleveland Clinic thus instituted Web-based business intelligence tools to provide clinicians with their performance data to engage them in quality improvement and waste reduction. This effort resulted in greater than 40% reduction in CLABSI and 50% reduction in CAUTI, with cost avoidances of $30,000 per CLABSI and $5000 per CAUTI.[26]

To increase the value of care for the surgical patient, the Perioperative Surgical Home must successfully translate, implement, and sustain these and other quality, safety, satisfaction improvement, and cost-reduction strategies in the perioperative continuum. Other examples include:

- Decrease practice variability, including unit of service cost for anesthesia services
- Increase practice efficiency, including the maximum use of advanced practice nurses
- Patient risk stratification and mitigation, including open dialogue about futile surgery
- Perioperative optimization of patient comorbidities, including optimal timing of surgery
- Patient education and counseling, including financial counseling before the day of surgery

THE PERIOPERATIVE SURGICAL HOME AS A NEW VALUE STREAM MAP

The basic philosophy and fundamentals of Lean methodology, derived from the Toyota Production System, can readily be applied in the health care environment, including in the acute hospital setting.[27] Lean in health care has been defined as "an organization's cultural commitment to applying the scientific method to designing, performing, and continuously improving the work delivered by teams of people, leading to measurably better value for patients and other stakeholders."[28] When applied effectively within the hospital setting, Lean can improve quality, patient safety, and employee engagement.[29]

There are 6 principles that constitute the essential dynamic of Lean management, which must all be embraced to fully realize the potential of Lean to benefit a health care organization's stakeholders,[28] including its ultimate customers—its patients:

- Attitude of continuous improvement
- Value creation
- Unity of purpose
- Respect for front-line workers
- Visual tracking
- Flexible regimentation

One of the most commonly used tools in Lean methodology is value stream mapping, which graphically displays the process of services or product delivery through the use of inputs, throughputs, and outputs.[30] Hines and Rich[31,32] have described 7 value stream mapping tools:

- Process activity mapping
- Supply chain responsiveness matrix
- Product variety funnel
- Quality filter mapping
- Forrester effect mapping
- Decision point analysis
- Overall structure maps

The Perioperative Surgical Home represents a new value stream map, which can be detailed using process activity mapping (**Fig. 3**). This perioperative process activity map includes all 4 phases of patient care (preoperative, intraoperative, immediately postoperative, and post-hospital discharge) and the respective multiple patient contact points.

At the University of Alabama at Birmingham, the authors have emphasized efforts to move as much patient management activity upstream to the preoperative phase, including consenting for interventional analgesic techniques performed on the day of surgery, and post-hospital discharge planning. A more formal preoperative clearance process for selected patients has also implemented. Patients who are identified in the surgical clinics via a simple, self-completed questionnaire as having 1 or more major comorbidities are not assigned a definitive surgery date until they have been evaluated, optimized, and cleared for anesthesia by the Preoperative Assessment, Consultation, and Treatment Clinic.

A PERIOPERATIVE PERSONALIZED CARE MATRIX

Developing clinical practice guidelines is a highly structured, labor-intensive process, involving a rigorous review and critical appraisal of the literature, multidisciplinary consultation, and grading of the resulting recommendations based on the quality of available evidence.[33] Nevertheless, persistently variable success has been experienced in translating even well-grounded national or professional clinical guidelines into local practice, including in the perioperative setting.[34,35] Persistent barriers to health care providers adopting such clinical practice guidelines include inadequate understanding, lack of agreement and perceived real-world practicality, concerns about loss of self-efficacy, low outcome expectations, and the inertia of existing practice.[36] Applicability can be enhanced by adapting clinical practice guidelines within the local context, and their acceptance can be improved by assessing barriers to their use.[37]

At the University of Alabama at Birmingham, the authors have achieved increased applicability and acceptance of clinical practice guideline goals with their Perioperative Risk Optimization and Management Planning Tool (PROMPT). A PROMPT is an amalgamation of evidence-based best practice and local clinician expertise and consensus. Representative topics for a perioperative PROMPT include anemia management, anticoagulants, nausea and vomiting, multimodal analgesia, delirium and cognitive dysfunction, myocardial injury after noncardiac surgery, obstructive sleep apnea, and intraoperative protective mechanical ventilation.[11]

In contrast to a PROMPT, an integrated care pathway is a detailed, task-orientated care plan that (1) delineates the essential elements in the care of all patients undergoing a specific surgical procedure (eg, total hip arthroplasty or total knee arthroplasty), and then (2) highlights and addresses any lack of process standardization and resulting inefficiencies and waste.[11,38,39]

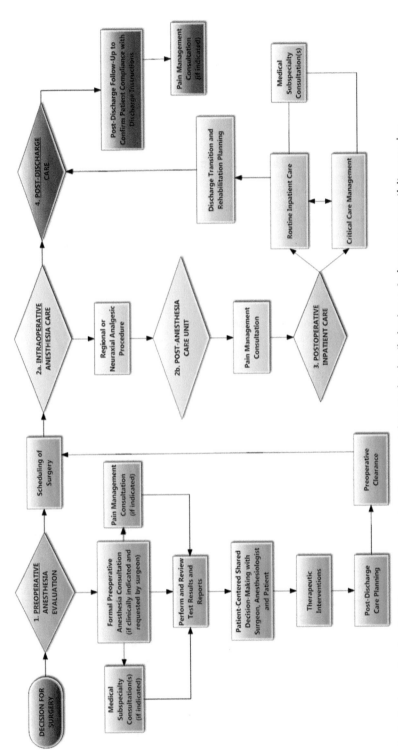

Fig. 3. Perioperative Surgical Home as a new value stream map that can be detailed using a 4-phase process activity mapping.

A PROMPT can complement and strengthen a surgical procedure–specific integrated care pathway. A patient-centric "perioperative personalized care matrix" can be created by the amalgamation of all of the standardized elements of a surgical procedure–specific integrated care pathway and any applicable condition–specific PROMPT (**Fig. 4**).[11] This perioperative personalized care matrix promotes the achievement of the IHI Triple Aim and delivery of patient-centered, value-based health care.

PYRAMID OF PRACTICE CHANGE: ROLE OF INFORMATICS, ANALYTICS, AND DECISION SUPPORT

The practice of medicine in the United States is undergoing a remarkable refocusing on how services are remunerated from the traditional fee-for-service model to one that is based predominately on the quality of care a health system provides to patients, families, and communities. Health care informatics, analytics, and decision support are the foundation and mechanisms for achieving practice change management. Informatics, analytics, and decision support collectively can be conceptually viewed as a pyramid of practice change (**Fig. 5**).

In addition to other key initiatives, health systems are making substantial investments in and use of health informatics as a key driver for change in models of care delivery to those that are less fragmented and more efficient, in part by making information more transparent and, thus, promoting accountability. Indeed, health informatics and the use of health information technology (HIT) have increasingly been identified as an essential component of the infrastructure and internal operational practices of high-reliability health care organizations.[40]

If designed properly and used consistently and effectively, HIT can be highly value-added by (1) increasing quality and patient safety, (2) promoting higher efficiency and more streamlined work processes, and (3) spurring lower cost and greater patient access to affordable care.[40] For example, HIT can provide real-time communication of information to and among health care professionals and care teams during the care

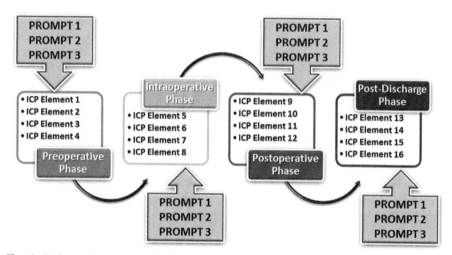

Fig. 4. Perioperative personalized care matrix. ICP, integrated care pathway; PROMPT, Perioperative Risk Optimization and Management Planning Tool. (*From* Vetter TR, Boudreaux AM, Jones KA, et al. The perioperative surgical home: how anesthesiology can collaboratively achieve and leverage the triple aim in health care. Anesth Analg 2014;118:1132; with permission.)

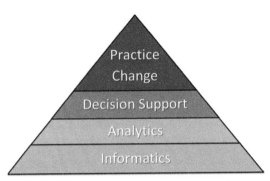

Fig. 5. Informatics, analytics, and decision support collectively form a pyramid of practice change.

process, thereby assisting in avoiding errors or improving compliance with evidence-informed care pathways. Furthermore, HIT can provide the umbrella infrastructure to comprehensively manage and provide secure information exchange between consumers, providers, governmental and other quality entities, and insurers.

As with high-reliability organizations, the use of health informatics is critical to the successful achievement of the tripartite or triple aim of the Perioperative Surgical Home. An essential element of the informatics capabilities of the Perioperative Surgical Home is the ability to fully integrate patient health information within the entire health system, including outpatient and inpatient point-of-service environments, with other data repositories such as laboratory and radiology, finance, quality metrics, and others.

Once data repositories are established and well connected, their rich, granular data can be extracted, coalesced, and analyzed, and the insights and knowledge gained can be used in decision making by patients, families, and health care providers. For example, such data can be used to develop real-time, front-line health informatics decision-support tools, which can be applied by the health care team in their day-to-day operations and facilitate patient-specific, personalized care planning, decisions, and implementation. Health information obtained during the preoperative phase of care can be used to identify patients' perioperative risk factors that can then be reliably communicated to all intraoperative and postoperative care providers. Also communicated to these providers are risk factor–based, evidence-informed protocols, which when consistently implemented could attenuate practice variability.

The development of these tools is best accomplished by the establishment of an interprofessional team of stakeholder clinicians who collaborate with information technology professionals to assess the information and knowledge needs of the health care professionals and their patients, and to characterize, evaluate, and refine clinical processes and the attendant decision-support systems. This team not only assesses the consistency with which the protocols are implemented but also measures and disseminates a predetermined scorecard of patient safety, quality of care, financial, and other metrics the protocols are purported to improve.

FUTURE CONSIDERATIONS AND SUMMARY

The Perioperative Surgical Home remains in its operational nascence. There will undoubtedly be multiple future and iterative variations of this concept that may work effectively, depending on local infrastructure and politics, in addition to known and yet to be identified internal and external forces.[11,25] However, to increase the value of care of the surgical patient, any Perioperative Surgical Home model must ultimately successfully translate, implement, and sustain quality, safety, and satisfaction improvement, and cost-reduction strategies in the perioperative continuum. Published outcomes data on the Perioperative Surgical Home models remain sparse. Hence, the timely data-based documenting and reporting of various institutional experiences is crucial.

REFERENCES

1. Sisko AM, Keehan SP, Cuckler GA, et al. National health expenditure projections, 2013-23: faster growth expected with expanded coverage and improving economy. Health Aff (Millwood) 2014;33:1841-50.
2. Health Care Cost Institute. Health care cost and utilization report. Washington, DC: Health Care Cost Institute; 2011-2012.
3. Cormier JN, Cromwell KD, Pollock RE. Value-based health care: a surgical oncologist's perspective. Surg Oncol Clin N Am 2012;21:497-506.
4. Fry DE, Pine M, Jones BL, et al. The impact of ineffective and inefficient care on the excess costs of elective surgical procedures. J Am Coll Surg 2011;212:779-86.
5. Vetter TR, Goeddel LA, Boudreaux AM, et al. The Perioperative Surgical Home: how can it make the case so everyone wins? BMC Anesthesiol 2013;13:6.
6. Stange KC, Nutting PA, Miller WL, et al. Defining and measuring the patient-centered medical home. J Gen Intern Med 2010;25:601-12.
7. Orszag PR, Emanuel EJ. Health care reform and cost control. N Engl J Med 2010; 363:601-3.
8. Fineberg HV. Shattuck lecture. A successful and sustainable health system—how to get there from here. N Engl J Med 2012;366:1020-7.
9. Berwick DM, Nolan TW, Whittington J. The triple aim: care, health, and cost. Health Aff (Millwood) 2008;27:759-69.
10. Stiefel M, Nolan K. A guide to measuring the triple aim: population health, experience of care, and per capita cost IHI innovation series white paper. Cambridge (MA): Institute for Healthcare Improvement; 2012.
11. Vetter TR, Boudreaux AM, Jones KA, et al. The perioperative surgical home: how anesthesiology can collaboratively achieve and leverage the triple aim in health care. Anesth Analg 2014;118:1131-6.
12. Cusack CM, Knudson AD, Kronstadt JL, et al. AHRQ National Resource Center for Health Information Technology. Practice-based population health: information technology to support transformation to proactive primary care. Rockville (MD): Agency for Healthcare Research and Quality; 2010.
13. Centers for Medicare and Medicaid Services. Readmissions reduction program. Baltimore (MD): Centers for Medicare and Medicaid Services; 2014.
14. Centers for Medicare and Medicaid Services. Hospital-acquired condition (HAC) reduction program. Baltimore (MD): Centers for Medicare and Medicaid Services; 2014.
15. Centers for Medicare and Medicaid Services. Hospital value-based purchasing. Baltimore (MD): Centers for Medicare and Medicaid Services; 2014.
16. QualityNet. Medicare spending per beneficiary (MSPB) measure overview. Baltimore (MD): Centers for Medicare and Medicaid Services; 2014.
17. Rajaram R, Barnard C, Bilimoria KY. Concerns about using the patient safety indicator-90 composite in pay-for-performance programs. JAMA 2015;313:897-8.
18. Barnes AJ, Unruh L, Chukmaitov A, et al. Accountable care organizations in the USA: types, developments and challenges. Health Policy 2014;118:1-7.

19. Muhlestein D. Continued growth of public and private accountable care organizations health affairs blog. Bethesda (MD): Project HOPE: The People-to-People Health Foundation, Inc; 2013.
20. Muhlestein D. Accountable care growth in 2014: a look ahead health affairs blog. Bethesda (MD): Project HOPE: The People-to-People Health Foundation, Inc; 2014.
21. Porter ME. What is value in health care? N Engl J Med 2010;363:2477–81.
22. Porter ME, Teisberg EO. Redefining health care: creating value-based competition on results. Boston: Harvard Business School Press; 2006.
23. Lee TH. Putting the value framework to work. N Engl J Med 2010;363:2481–3.
24. Porter ME, Pabo EA, Lee TH. Redesigning primary care: a strategic vision to improve value by organizing around patients' needs. Health Aff (Millwood) 2013;32:516–25.
25. Vetter TR, Ivankova NV, Goeddel LA, et al. An analysis of methodologies that can be used to validate if a Perioperative Surgical Home improves the patient-centeredness, evidence-based practice, quality, safety, and value of patient care. Anesthesiology 2013;119:1261–74.
26. Cosgrove D, Fisher M, Gabow P, et al. A CEO checklist for high-value health care. Washington, DC: Institute of Medicine; 2012.
27. Kim CS, Spahlinger DA, Kin JM, et al. Lean health care: what can hospitals learn from a world-class automaker? J Hosp Med 2006;1:191–9.
28. Toussaint JS, Berry LL. The promise of Lean in health care. Mayo Clin Proc 2013;88:74–82.
29. Graban M. Lean hospitals: improving quality, patient safety, and employee engagement. Boca Raton (FL): CRC Press; 2012.
30. Varkey P, Reller MK, Resar RK. Basics of quality improvement in health care. Mayo Clin Proc 2007;82:735–9.
31. Hines, Peter, Rich N. The seven value stream mapping tools. Int J Oper Prod Man 1997;17(1):46–64.
32. Rich N, Bateman N, Esain A, et al. Understanding your organisation lean evolution: lessons from the workplace. Cambridge (United Kingdom): Cambridge University Press; 2006. p. 32–59.
33. Woolf S, Schunemann HJ, Eccles MP, et al. Developing clinical practice guidelines: types of evidence and outcomes; values and economics, synthesis, grading, and presentation and deriving recommendations. Implement Sci 2012;7:61.
34. Bosse G, Breuer JP, Spies C. The resistance to changing guidelines—what are the challenges and how to meet them. Best Pract Res Clin Anaesthesiol 2006;20:379–95.
35. Vetter TR, Hunter JM Jr, Boudreaux AM. Preoperative management of antiplatelet drugs for a coronary artery stent: how can we hit a moving target? BMC Anesthesiol 2014;14:73.
36. Cabana MD, Rand CS, Powe NR, et al. Why don't physicians follow clinical practice guidelines? A framework for improvement. JAMA 1999;282:1458–65.
37. Harrison MB, Legare F, Graham ID, et al. Adapting clinical practice guidelines to local context and assessing barriers to their use. CMAJ 2010;182:E78–84.
38. Campbell H, Hotchkiss R, Bradshaw N, et al. Integrated care pathways. BMJ 1998;316:133–7.
39. Napolitano LM. Standardization of perioperative management: clinical pathways. Surg Clin North Am 2005;85:1321–7.
40. Chaudhry B, Wang J, Wu S, et al. Systematic review: impact of health information technology on quality, efficiency, and costs of medical care. Ann Intern Med 2006;144:742–52.

The Pain Medical Home
A Patient-Centered Medical Home Model
of Care for Patients with Chronic Pain

Peter Pryzbylkowski, MD*, Michael A. Ashburn, MD, MPH

KEYWORDS

- Patient-centered medical home • Collaborative care • Chronic pain
- Interdisciplinary pain management • Value-based care

KEY POINTS

- Chronic pain costs society anywhere from $560 to $635 billion a year.
- Patients with pain typically have multiple coexisting medical and psychiatric conditions that make adequate control of their pain symptoms difficult.
- The use of opioids for the treatment of chronic pain has increased significantly over the last 2 decades, in spite of very limited data supporting efficacy and clear evidence of significant risk of harm, including death.
- Integrated, interdisciplinary pain care has been advocated for decades, as there is clear evidence that this model of care is associated with improved patient outcomes. However, there are several barriers to providing this type of care to patients with chronic pain.
- The patient-centered medical home model of care presents an opportunity to improve patient outcomes through improved coordination of care among the care team, including the primary care physician.

INTRODUCTION

Chronic pain is a common disorder for which patients seek care from a variety of health care providers. In addition to chronic pain, these patients often also suffer from depression, sleep disturbance, fatigue, and overall poor mental and physical

The authors would both like to disclose that they have no financial conflicts of interest in relationship to the creation of this article.
Department of Anesthesiology and Critical Care, University of Pennsylvania, Philadelphia, PA, USA
* Corresponding author. Penn Pain Medicine Center, 1840 South Street, Philadelphia, PA 19035.
E-mail address: Peter.Pryzbylkowski@uphs.upenn.edu

Anesthesiology Clin 33 (2015) 785–793
http://dx.doi.org/10.1016/j.anclin.2015.07.009   **anesthesiology.theclinics.com**
1932-2275/15/$ – see front matter © 2015 Elsevier Inc. All rights reserved.

functioning. Although there are significant gaps in the evidence supporting several pain treatment options, there is clear evidence that integrated, interdisciplinary care leads to improved outcomes.[1] Unfortunately, such care is often unavailable or, if available, barriers often exist to prevent individual patients from accessing this interdisciplinary care.

Patients with chronic pain often seek care for their condition through their primary care physician. However, primary care physicians may not have the resources available to properly diagnose and treat many chronic pain conditions. Specialty care may be available, but identifying the proper specialist and coordinating this care can be very difficult. As a result, the care of patients with complex chronic pain often ends up fragmented among several providers who may provide care absent careful coordination of this care among all involved providers.

This review of chronic pain care will explore the following:

- Current evidence-based approaches to caring for patients with chronic pain
- The role of interdisciplinary clinics and establishment of a pain medical home
- How pain clinics add value to the health care system

The financial burden that chronic pain places on our society is staggering. The combined cost of health care utilization and decreased productivity from chronic pain ranges from $560 to $635 billion annually. Although this number has been criticized for possibly being too high, others have reported that this may be a conservative estimate and the real cost of chronic pain to society may actually be much higher.[2]

Chronic pain affects more Americans than diabetes, heart disease, and cancer combined, with 2011 estimates of 116 million adults being affected.[3] Chronic pain includes the pain associated with chronic painful conditions, such as arthritis, as well as painful conditions in which the underlying causes of pain may not be clear. Chronic pain often includes abnormal neuropathic pain states, which are often associated with nerve damage following trauma or surgery.

Chronic back pain is the most prevalent chronic pain condition, and chronic low back pain is a major cause for increased health care utilization and decreased workforce productivity.[4,5] Evidence-based guidelines regarding the treatment of low back pain exist,[6] but their impact on the process of patient care is unclear. Likewise, studies have shown that multidisciplinary clinics that treat low back pain have better outcomes than those who only provide one treatment modality; however, these clinics are currently few and far between.[7] As is seen throughout the United States health care system, chronic pain care is provided in a highly variable manner, and coordination of care is often lacking. Patient outcomes likely can be improved through improvements in the process of care, especially if patient outcomes are used to guide process improvement efforts.

THE PATIENT-CENTERED MEDICAL HOME

The patient-centered medical home (PCMH) model of care was described in 2008 by the American College of Physicians and the American Academy of Family Physicians.[8] This model of care was developed to improve patient satisfaction and health care outcomes, with a focus of improving the process of care in the primary care setting. This model of care focuses on providing integrated, team-based care, and encourages care teams to leverage technology to develop innovative solutions toward effective communications with patients and among team members.

> The following are features of the PCMH:
>
> Personal physician: Each patient has an ongoing relationship with a personal physician who provides first contact along with continuous and comprehensive care.
>
> Physician-directed medical practice: The personal physician leads a team of individuals at the practice level that collectively assume the responsibility of patient care.
>
> Whole-person orientation: The personal physician is responsible for providing the patients' entire health care needs or arranging this care with qualified professionals.
>
> Coordinated care: Health care is provided in an integrated and coordinated manner across all elements of the health care system.
>
> Evidence-based care: A focus on quality and safety is a hallmark of the medical home, with patients actively participating in medical decision making and practitioners using evidence-based medicine to guide clinical decision making.
>
> Innovative solutions: The health care team uses innovative solutions to provide enhanced access to proper care, such as open-access scheduling, expanded hours, and new options for communication (eg, e-consults) between patients, their personal physician, and practice staff.

Of note, when the PCMH model of care was originally described, there was no mention of integrating behavioral health services into the model. This point is important because, as discussed previously, many patients with chronic pain have behavioral health issues. Recently, this issue has been addressed by psychiatric specialists that are now trying to incorporate behavioral health services into the PCMH model of care.[9] This task is important because behavioral health is tightly interwoven with physical well-being and overall health outcomes are improved when behavioral health issues are integrated and treated in the primary care setting.[10]

PATIENT-CENTERED MEDICAL HOME-NEIGHBOR

The PCMH model of care was expanded to include specialty care through the development of the PCMH-neighbor (PCMH-N). The PCMH-N outlines the roles that specialty providers serve in patient care. The Council of Subspecialty Societies of the American College of Physicians endorsed this model of care. The council recognizes specialty/subspecialty practices as a PCMH-N if they engage in the following[11]:

- Ensure effective communication, coordination, and integration with PCMH practices in a bidirectional manner to provide high-quality and efficient care
- Ensure appropriate and timely consultations and referrals
- Ensure the efficient, appropriate, and effective flow of necessary patient and care information
- Effectively guide determination of responsibility in comanagement situations
- Support patient-centered care, enhanced care access, and high levels of care quality and safety
- Support the PCMH practice as the provider of whole-person primary care to patients and as having overall responsibility for ensuring the coordination and integration of the care provided by all involved physicians and other health care professionals

Thus, the emphasis of the PCMH-N process of care is efficient, timely patient care associated with efficient, timely communication and coordination of care between the specialist and primary care physician.

Technology provides opportunities for innovative solutions regarding improving the process of communication and coordination of care, including care interactions by providers with patients and their families. These technologies include electronic referral and consult management,[12] telemedicine,[13] and treatment-specific specialty education classes.[14] Creation of efficient medical neighborhoods will most likely require an expanded framework that includes a broader array of interaction types that relies more heavily on advancements in technology.[15]

THE PAIN MEDICAL HOME

The pain medical home represents an attempt to bring the concepts of the PCMH model of care into play for patients with chronic pain. This article focuses on efforts to improve the process of care provided by the primary care team and the pain specialists but can also apply to other specialists involved in the care of patients with chronic pain.

Care using the PCMH approach emphasizes the importance of integrated, interdisciplinary care. It is important to note that integrated interdisciplinary care has been a cornerstone of chronic pain care for decades. Therefore, this process of care is clearly not a new creation but rather a reinvigoration of a concept originally advocated by John Bonica[16] and others.

Initial efforts regarding the development and implementation of a pain medical home has been focused on the subpopulation of patients with chronic pain requiring chronic opioids as part of their pain treatment. However, such a model can also easily be used for other chronic pain conditions, including chronic low back pain.

As discussed earlier, core concepts of the PCMH include the presence of a personal physician, the use of a physician-directed medical practice team, a whole-person orientation to care, and careful coordination of care. Additional concepts related to the integration of specialty care include sharing a common vision for the care process, careful delineation of the roles and responsibilities for team members, the importance of timely referrals, and timely and efficient communication among team members. By way of example, the authors briefly describe their experience using the PCMH-N model of care to develop a process of care related to the use of opioids to treat chronic pain at the University of Pennsylvania.

Shared Vision

It is difficult to build effective teams, and such teams require that team members share a common vision for what the team hopes to accomplish. This common vision can only occur following the development of an understanding of the skills and interests of key team members and the development of mutual trust and respect. A shared vision includes the joint development of the process of care that is evidence-based and takes into account the resources and capabilities of team members. Clearly, the process of care cannot be developed by one member of the team absent open collaboration from other team members.

When a decision was made to explore the opportunity to improve the process of care related to the use of opioids to treat chronic pain, an integrated team was developed. This team included physician leadership, physicians, nurse practitioners, and support staff of the involved primary care practice. In addition, physician leadership, physicians, psychologists, and support staff of the involved pain specialty practice were on the team. This team met on a regular basis and documented the projects goals and then jointly outlined a process of care and communication among team members, with a focus toward improving patient outcomes.

Personal Physician

As part of the shared vision development, the important role of the primary care physician in the patient care team needs to be recognized and maintained. Specialty care team members must recognize the importance of making every effort to ensure that the primary care physician is actively involved in ongoing patient care, including weighing in on important health care decisions. The role of the primary care physician in ongoing care should be emphasized by specialty team members.

With regard to the chronic opioid process, the leadership role of the primary care physician was recognized and integrated into the process of care. The pain specialty team does not start chronic opioid therapy until a formal collaborative agreement between the pain specialist and the primary care physician is in place. This agreement documents the roles that each team will play during the provision of care and also documents the core concepts of care that will be used during chronic opioid therapy (such as regular visits, no early opioid refills, regular urine drug screens, and the process for monitoring the patients' response to therapy). A process for clear communication among team members was established, including a process to clearly document which team will be responsible for prescribing opioids.

Evidence-Based Care

Outcomes are optimized when the process of care is based on best evidence whenever possible. However, a standardized process of care, even when evidence is limited to guide decision making, will reduce the variability of care and improve outcomes. In addition, a standardized approach will allow for all team members, including support staff, to anticipate the next steps in the process of care and avoid preventable treatment errors. Care must be taken to consider available resources and limitations, so that unreasonable expectations are not established.

Careful Delineation of Roles and Responsibilities

The process of care should be diagrammed and outlined, and team member roles and responsibilities should be clearly identified. Special attention should be paid to transitions in care, as care transitions present unique challenges to ensure effective communication among team members; all team members need to be aware when they assume responsibility for a specific activity related to patient care.

Careful Coordination of Care

When new teams are created, members often identify opportunities for improvements in team communication. Care should be taken to develop and implement a process of care that ensures timely, effective communication among team members. Consideration should be given to the creation of regular meetings of team leadership to discuss problems as they arise to allow for process improvement efforts as learning occurs.

With regard to the chronic opioid project, the integrated team reviewed existing evidence-based guidelines regarding the use of chronic opioids to treat noncancer pain and developed a standardized process of care based on the guidelines and practice-specific conditions. It was then the responsibility of each individual practice to implement and monitor compliance with the established process of care.

Physician-Directed Care Team

Both the primary care team and the pain specialty care teams include physician and nonphysician providers. Key members of the pain specialty team include the pain psychologist, physical therapist, and nurse, among others. As has been described earlier, the pain specialty team should share a common vision for care and provide integrated, interdisciplinary care in cooperation with the primary care team.

Focus on the Person Rather than the Disease

Patients with chronic pain can be expected to be experiencing pain in combination with changes in mood, sleep, and compromise of physical and mental functioning. These health conditions often adversely impact family and work life, and as a result significant stress is present. Patients with pain often have 1 or more comorbid health conditions, including conditions associated with advancing age. As a result, care often must include coordinated care from multiple providers, attending the risk of possible drug-drug interactions as well as an increased risk for adverse events. Care should often include medication therapy, activating physical therapy, cognitive-behavioral therapy, and interventional therapy.

Innovative Solutions

Timely, rich communication between patients and their family, as well as among care team members, is often made possible through the use of innovative solutions. These solutions include the establishment of a standard process to document care and communicate within the electronic health record, innovative scheduling to allow for efficient use of limited health care resources, timely interactions between patients and members of the health care team, and the use of novel communication methods, including e-mail, texting, and Internet-based patient education. In addition, electronic data capture can allow for collection and tracking of patient-reported outcome measures as well as the establishment and tracking of goals of treatment, documenting shared decision making between patients and the health care team.

THE IMPORTANCE OF ASSESSING OUTCOMES IN THE PAIN MEDICAL HOME

Even though major advances have occurred in pain medicine over the past 30 years, chronic pain is often poorly controlled. The fact still remains that there is no good, robust evidence-based medicine to help guide the clinician in the treatment of patients with chronic pain. The lack of solid evidence-based medicine for chronic pain leads to the poor results that are typically seen with patients with chronic pain.

Therefore, it is especially important for the pain medical home to collect outcomes data so that information gathered during patient treatment can be used to guide care and improve treatment outcomes. Typically for patients with chronic pain the most commonly used outcome measure is patient-reported pain intensity. However, for these patients, it is also important to measure their physical and mental well-being as well as patient satisfaction with the care they receive.[17] Patient pain outcomes can be improved through the standardization of the process of patient care as well as through other quality improvement efforts. Efforts to improve patient pain outcomes should be an ongoing process that is fluid and allows the pain medical home to show its value in providing high quality care for its patients.[18] The quality in care provided can be tracked by measurement of meaningful pain outcome data over time; these data can then be used to show value for services provided.

WHERE IS THE PAIN MEDICAL HOME?

There is still debate as to where the patient pain medical home should be (at the primary care level vs under supervision of pain specialist). No matter where the leadership of the home is, it is apparent that the pain medical home should encompass a team that is cohesive and brings with it a multimodal approach to treating pain. In the Veterans Affairs (VA) Connecticut Healthcare System, the interdisciplinary pain care team has been introduced at the level of the primary care physician. The VA was able to introduce both an integrated pain clinic and opioid reassessment clinic that is embedded within primary care services. The creation of these 2 separate resources led to higher rates of engagement in specialty and multimodal pain care services along with both higher provider and patient satisfaction with the care provided.[19]

Although the participation of pain specialists can add significant resources, the process of providing chronic pain care can be improved even when such specialty care is not available. Chronic pain care poses similar issues to treatment that other chronic disorders, such as diabetes, present to care teams. In New Mexico, a new model of health care education and delivery called Project ECHO (Extension for Community Healthcare Outcomes) has been shown to provide quality primary and specialty care to a rural underserved patient population, even when access to specialty care is limited. This new health care model has successfully taught primary care physicians how to treat patients with chronic hepatitis C through the aid of telemedicine grand rounds and case presentations. During these telemedicine talks, the primary care providers can discuss cases with other general practice providers and gain guidance from liver specialists from the University of New Mexico who participate in the online conferences. Primary care providers reported major benefits from taking part in the program and reported increased competence in their ability to assess, treat, and manage patients with hepatitis C.[20] Clearly, similar innovative processes of care could be used to improve chronic pain care.

As technological advances continue and allow providers to speak with specialists in large academic medical centers to improve care, chronic pain patients can also take advantage of these advances. In a study of chronic musculoskeletal pain, patients randomized to undergo telecare management of their symptoms through a pain specialist/primary care provider versus treatment as usual through the primary care provider had better pain scores at 12 months and reported at least a 30% improvement in their pain during the study period.[21]

SUMMARY AND FUTURE CONSIDERATIONS

Chronic pain continues to affect millions of Americans and costs our society billions of dollars a year.[3] To this day, treatment of patients with chronic pain is difficult, costly, and nonintegrative. Patients with chronic pain are difficult to treat; hence, outcomes are poor because they tend to present with comorbidities (undiagnosed major psychiatric issues and/or sleep disturbances) that make it hard to treat their pain effectively with medications, including opioids. Pain care and how it is currently being delivered in this country needs to be rethought. We can no longer continue to provide care that does not provide meaningful benefit and substantial outcomes to the patients we treat.

The patient-centered pain medical home as it is described in this article is the exception rather than the norm in our country. It is a model of care that is not well reimbursed; hence, it is a model that is not feasible for most pain practices or providers. Until this model is well reimbursed, care for patients with chronic pain will continue to be fraught with poor outcomes. This article reviews the benefits of a pain medical home, including the coordination of care among multiple providers, the benefits of integrative care in restoring patient function, and the money that can be saved over time from a comprehensive pain treatment approach. As always, the integrative model of care that is provided by the pain medical home relies on constant communication between providers and, even more importantly, on communication with the general practitioner.

No matter what setting pain care is provided in, it is very important to measure outcome data. No longer is it appropriate to provide medications, such as opioids, that have the potential to cause tremendous harm to patients if meaningful outcomes are not being tracked and followed over time. Once outcome data are generated, it will be easier to perform meaningful research that will help provide further evidence for treatment of patients with chronic pain. As it currently stands, high-quality evidence supporting chronic pain management is few and far between.

REFERENCES

1. Ashburn MA, Staats PS. Management of chronic pain. Lancet 1999;353(9167): 1865–9.
2. Gaskin DJ, Richard P. The economic costs of pain in the United States. J Pain 2012;13(8):715–24.
3. Pizzo, Clark, Carter-Pokras, et al. Relieving pain in America: a blueprint for transforming prevention, care, education, and research. Washington, DC: The National Academies Press; 2011.
4. Breivik H, Collett B, Ventafridda V, et al. Survey of chronic pain in Europe: prevalence, impact on daily life, and treatment. Eur J Pain 2006;10(4):287–333.
5. Becker A. Health economics of interdisciplinary rehabilitation for chronic pain: does it support or invalidate the outcomes research of these programs? Curr Pain Headache Rep 2012;16(2):127–32.
6. Chou R. In the clinic. Low back pain. Ann Intern Med 2014;160(11):ITC6-1.
7. Flor H, Fydrich T, Turk DC. Efficacy of multidisciplinary pain treatment centers: a meta-analytic review. Pain 1992;49(2):221–30.
8. American Academy of Family Physicians. Joint principles of the patient-centered medical home. Del Med J 2008;80(1):21–2.
9. Working Party Group on Integrated Behavioral Healthcare, Baird M, Blount A, et al. Joint principles: integrating behavioral health care into the patient-centered medical home. Ann Fam Med 2014;12(2):183–5.
10. Anderson NB, Belar CD, Cubic BA, et al. Statement of the American Psychological Association in response to the "joint principles: integrating behavioral health care into the patient-centered medical home". Fam Syst Health 2014;32(2): 141–2.
11. Greenlee MC, Honsinger R, Kirschner N. The patient-centered medical home neighbor. Ann Intern Med 2011;154(11):779–80.
12. Chen AH, Kushel MB, Grumbach K, et al. Practice profile. A safety-net system gains efficiencies through 'eReferrals' to specialists. Health Aff 2010;29(5): 969–71.
13. Bashshur RL, Shannon GW, Krupinski EA, et al. National telemedicine initiatives: essential to healthcare reform. Telemed J E Health 2009;15(6):600–10.
14. Surjadi M, Torruellas C, Ayala C, et al. Formal patient education improves patient knowledge of hepatitis C in vulnerable populations. Dig Dis Sci 2011;56(1):213–9.
15. Yee HF Jr. The patient-centered medical home neighbor: a subspecialty physician's view. Ann Intern Med 2011;154(1):63–4.
16. Bonica JJ. Basic principles in managing chronic pain. Arch Surg 1977;112(6): 783–8.
17. Gupta A, Ashburn M, Ballantyne J. Quality assurance and assessment in pain management. Anesthesiol Clin 2011;29(1):123–33.
18. Witkin LR, Farrar JT, Ashburn MA. Can assessing chronic pain outcomes data improve outcomes? Pain Med 2013;14(6):779–91.

19. Dorflinger LM, Ruser C, Sellinger J, et al. Integrating interdisciplinary pain management into primary care: development and implementation of a novel clinical program. Pain Med 2014;15(12):2046-54.
20. Arora S, Kalishman S, Dion D, et al. Partnering urban academic medical centers and rural primary care clinicians to provide complex chronic disease care. Health Aff 2011;30(6):1176-84.
21. Kroenke K, Krebs EE, Wu J, et al. Telecare collaborative management of chronic pain in primary care: a randomized clinical trial. JAMA 2014;312(3):240-8.

Index

Anesthesiology Clin 33 (2015) 795–803
http://dx.doi.org/10.1016/S1932-2275(15)00101-9
1932-2275/15/$ – see front matter © 2015 Elsevier Inc. All rights reserved.

United States Postal Service

Statement of Ownership, Management, and Circulation
(All Periodicals Publications Except Requestor Publications)

1. Publication Title	2. Publication Number	3. Filing Date
Anesthesiology Clinics	0 0 0 0 - 2 7 7 7	9/18/15

4. Issue Frequency	5. Number of Issues Published Annually	6. Annual Subscription Price
Mar, Jun, Sep, Dec	4	$330.00

7. Complete Mailing Address of Known Office of Publication (Not printer) (Street, city, county, state, and ZIP+4®)

Elsevier Inc.
360 Park Avenue South
New York, NY 10010-1710

Contact Person
Stephen R. Bushing

Telephone (Include area code)
215-239-3688

8. Complete Mailing Address of Headquarters or General Business Office of Publisher (Not printer)

Elsevier Inc., 360 Park Avenue South, New York, NY 10010-1710

9. Full Names and Complete Mailing Addresses of Publisher, Editor, and Managing Editor (Do not leave blank)

Publisher (Name and complete mailing address)

Linda Belfus, Elsevier Inc., 1600 John F. Kennedy Blvd., Suite 1800, Philadelphia, PA 19103

Editor (Name and complete mailing address)

Patrick Manley, Elsevier Inc., 1600 John F. Kennedy Blvd., Suite 1800, Philadelphia, PA 19103-2899

Managing Editor (Name and complete mailing address)

Adrianne Brigido, Elsevier Inc., 1600 John F. Kennedy Blvd., Suite 1800, Philadelphia, PA 19103-2899

10. Owner (Do not leave blank. If the publication is owned by a corporation, give the name and address of the corporation immediately followed by the names and addresses of all stockholders owning or holding 1 percent or more of the total amount of stock. If not owned by a corporation, give the names and addresses of the individual owners. If owned by a partnership or other unincorporated firm, give its name and address as well as those of each individual owner. If the publication is published by a nonprofit organization, give its name and address.)

Full Name	Complete Mailing Address
Wholly owned subsidiary of	1600 John F. Kennedy Blvd, Ste. 1800
Reed/Elsevier, US holdings	Philadelphia, PA 19103-2899

11. Known Bondholders, Mortgagees, and Other Security Holders Owning or Holding 1 Percent or More of Total Amount of Bonds, Mortgages, or Other Securities. If none, check box ☐ None

Full Name	Complete Mailing Address
N/A	

12. Tax Status (For completion by nonprofit organizations authorized to mail at nonprofit rates) (Check one)
The purpose, function, and nonprofit status of this organization and the exempt status for federal income tax purposes:
☐ Has Not Changed During Preceding 12 Months
☐ Has Changed During Preceding 12 Months (Publisher must submit explanation of change with this statement)

13. Publication Title	14. Issue Date for Circulation Data Below
Anesthesiology Clinics	September 2015

15. Extent and Nature of Circulation			Average No. Copies Each Issue During Preceding 12 Months	No. Copies of Single Issue Published Nearest to Filing Date
a. Total Number of Copies (Net press run)			755	614
b. Legitimate Paid and/Or Requested Distribution (By Mail and Outside the Mail)	(1)	Mailed Outside-County Paid/Requested Mail Subscriptions stated on PS Form 3541. (Include paid distribution above nominal rate, advertiser's proof copies and exchange copies)	240	156
	(2)	Mailed In-County Paid/Requested Mail Subscriptions stated on PS Form 3541. (Include paid distribution above nominal rate, advertiser's proof copies and exchange copies)		
	(3)	Paid Distribution Outside the Mails Including Sales Through Dealers And Carriers, Street Vendors, Counter Sales, and Other Paid Distribution Outside USPS®	200	242
	(4)	Paid Distribution by Other Classes of Mail Through the USPS (e.g. First-Class Mail®)		
c. Total Paid and/or Requested Circulation (Sum of 15b (1), (2), (3), and (4))		▲	440	398
d. Free or Nominal Rate Distribution (By Mail and Outside the Mail)	(1)	Free or Nominal Rate Outside-County Copies included on PS Form 3541	78	71
	(2)	Free or Nominal Rate In-County Copies included on PS Form 3541		
	(3)	Free or Nominal Rate Copies mailed at Other classes Through the USPS (e.g. First-Class Mail®)		
	(4)	Free or Nominal Rate Distribution Outside the Mail (Carriers or Other means)		
e. Total Nonrequested Distribution (Sum of 15d (1), (2), (3) and (4))			78	71
f. Total Distribution (Sum of 15c and 15e)		▲	518	469
g. Copies not Distributed (See instructions to publishers #4 (page #3))		▲	237	145
h. Total (Sum of 15f and g)		▲	755	614
i. Percent Paid and/or Requested Circulation (15c divided by 15f times 100)			84.94%	84.86%

* If you are claiming electronic copies go to line 16 on page 3. If you are not claiming
Electronic copies, skip to line 17 on page 3.

16. Electronic Copy Circulation	Average No. Copies Each Issue During Preceding 12 Months	No. Copies of Single Issue Published Nearest to Filing Date
a. Paid Electronic Copies		
b. Total paid Print Copies (Line 15c) + Paid Electronic copies (Line 16a)		
c. Total Print Distribution (Line 15f) + Paid Electronic Copies (Line 16a)		
d. Percent Paid (Both Print & Electronic copies) (16b divided by 16c X 100)		

☐ I certify that 50% of all my distributed copies (electronic and print) are paid above a nominal price

17. Publication of Statement of Ownership
If the publication is a general publication, publication of this statement is required. Will be printed in the __December 2015__ issue of this publication.

18. Signature and Title of Editor, Publisher, Business Manager, or Owner

Stephen R. Bushing

Stephen R. Bushing – Inventory Distribution Coordinator

Date
September 18, 2015

I certify that all information furnished on this form is true and complete. I understand that anyone who furnishes false or misleading information on this form or who omits material or information requested on the form may be subject to criminal sanctions (including fines and imprisonment) and/or civil sanctions (including civil penalties).

PS Form 3526, July 2014 (Page 3 of 3)

PS Form 3526, July 2014 (Page 1 of 3 (Instructions Page 3)) (Instructions Page 3)) PSN 7530-01-000-9931 PRIVACY NOTICE: See our Privacy policy in www.usps.com

Moving?

Make sure your subscription moves with you!

To notify us of your new address, find your **Clinics Account Number** (located on your mailing label above your name), and contact customer service at:

Email: journalscustomerservice-usa@elsevier.com

800-654-2452 (subscribers in the U.S. & Canada)
314-447-8871 (subscribers outside of the U.S. & Canada)

Fax number: 314-447-8029

Elsevier Health Sciences Division
Subscription Customer Service
3251 Riverport Lane
Maryland Heights, MO 63043

Printed and bound by CPI Group (UK) Ltd, Croydon, CR0 4YY

08/06/2025

01896870-0015